Health Savings Accounts
Planning for Prosperity

George Ross Fisher, MD

Ross & Perry Book Publishers
3 South Haddon Avenue
Haddonfield, New Jersey 08033
856-427-6135

George Ross Fisher MD

Also by the same author:
The Hospital That Ate Chicago, Saunders Press, 1980
Health Saving Accounts: A Handbook, Ross & Perry, Inc. 2015 *(Forthcoming)*

Copyright: 1-2540412791

ISBN #: 978-1-931839-44-0

Ross & Perry Book Publishers
3 South Haddon Avenue
Haddonfield, New Jersey 08033
856-427-6135

Acknowledgements

For advice and support about the thrust of this book, I owe spiritual debts to John McClaughry of Vermont, the late F. Michael Smith, Jr. of Louisiana, and the late Bill Niskanen of Minnesota and Washington, DC. It's heartening to remember strong support coming from wide corners of America, and from strata of society ranging from a country doctor, to the former Chairman of the President's Council of Economic Advisors. All three of these men worked their way up to being either a candidate for Governor of his state, the President of his State Medical Society, or the Chairman of a famous Washington think-tank. All three brushed aside the problems they created for themselves by constantly thinking outside of the box. My fellow Philadelphian John Bogle, whom I have only fleetingly met twice, deserves a lot of credit for demonstrating in his books how to invent a complicated concept, and then simplify it for outsiders. I've adopted his investing strategy.

And for personal support and tolerance from my family editorial board, consisting of my two sons and two daughters. My son George took time out from climbing the tallest mountains in the world, to develop a computer algorithm that instantly created the answers to a multitude of math problems hidden in certain assertions I blithely make, but now have confidence in. Likewise, my CPA daughter Miriam, told me some things which may be commonplace among corporate Chief Financial Officers, but astonish the rest of us. And her siblings Stuart and Margaret, who understood my tendency to wise-crack, but having long practice with its consequences, talked me out of most of it. Especially Margaret, who persuaded me it was more important for the title to be accurate, than to be witty.

Table of Contents

SECTION ONE

Health Savings Accounts
and its Competitor, in Brief

Health Savings Accounts and its Competitor, in Brief

Introduction

This book, a series of expansions on the Health Savings Account idea, is written in 2015 by one of its 1980 originators. It has been revised and rewritten several times, only to have a development or Court decision force it into yet another revision. After the United States Supreme Court decision of *King v. Burwell*, I decided to make one hurried revision and then stop revising it. It had grown to five hundred pages, well past the length the public would tolerate without a total rewrite, so it was severely cut, with the plan to take the excised pieces and bring them out separately as *Handbook of Health Savings Accounts.* I hope to produce the latter book soon, but it cannot be promised. This one, with still a few ragged edges, is written for the public and the Congress in order to have the main issues become part of the coming debate. I hope some of its editorial defects from the cutting process can be overlooked.

The Difference Between the Two Plans Let's get started right away, with a short simple summary of the two plans. It's one that everyone would agree is a simplification. The Affordable Care Act, universally described as Obamacare, is essentially the same as the employer-based health insurance we had for a century, with the main difference, it is intended to be universal and mandatory. By making it mandatory, it has to be subsidized for poor people. To pay for the subsidy, it has to be mandatory, because mandatory premiums on healthy uninsured are mostly used to pay for poor sick people. So, in spite of its title, it was destined to be expensive from the start.

Health Savings Accounts, on the other hand, are owned by the individual, and any savings are his to keep. Only high-deductible

("Catastrophic") costs are insured, and small-cost health costs are included only to the extent the individual chooses to include them, so naturally they are inherently cheaper. If he is shrewd and overfunds them, however, he can collect interest income which will reduce costs in the long future, – and if he doesn't spend the money on health, it is available to spend in his retirement. It has no mandatory links to the employer, so the problems caused by employer linkage are absent. That would include pre-existing conditions, job-lock, and gaps in coverage between employers. In thirty years, no one has successfully challenged the assertion they are cheaper. And by their design, it is hard to see why they wouldn't be cheaper. True, they don't cover the poor, but if the same government subsidy were to be applied to Health Savings Accounts as they are to Obamacare, the poor would be just as covered by HSA as by ACA. There you are, with a summary for late comers of the main differences between them. Two things were unexpected, however.

> In the first place, no one really expected Obamacare, for all its claim of universal coverage, would leave thirty million people uninsured. They can be summarized as seven million prisoners in custody, eight million disabled, and eleven million illegal aliens.

> And in the second place, no one really anticipated the investment income from Health Savings Accounts would compound to such large amounts. That comes from the greatly increased longevity, which allows compound interest to multiply mightily before the individual finally gets sick and uses the money. There are dozens of other small differences between the two plans, but this seems to me to be a fair summary for those who don't want to get down into the weeds, as politicians say. If you read the whole book, I feel most people would say this was a fair, rough, summary of its narrative. But as I went along, I added some new ideas. Most readers will find five or six really innovative ideas, which even I did not expect to discover.

Most of the Republican candidates for President have included classical HSA in their campaign platforms, but necessarily cannot endorse expanded versions without reading them. However, this is not a political book and fifteen million satisfied subscribers have already enrolled in the classical version. The Lifetime version requires serious legislation, suggested here in detail, but only as a goal.

Following two unexpected Supreme Court decisions, a third, revised, version called New Health Savings Accounts (N-HSA) was added, covering the 68% of healthcare costs not covered by the Affordable Care Act, but not particularly in conflict with it, either. If the two political parties could agree to compromise, pieces of these proposals might be useful in the debates. However, the economics of that proposal proved too precarious in the present vexed climate. The final version

> - C HSA (Classical)
> - L HSA (Lifetime)
> - N HSA (New)
>
> **Health Savings Accounts**

of N-HSA will however come as a surprise, consisting of pieces developing slowly as the book progressed, and centering on two entirely new concepts: the first year of life and the last year of life. Since they affect 100% of the population, they contribute much more to costs than any individual disease. Consequently, their main cost effect is implicit; taking them separately lowers the cost of other healthcare programs which overlap them. Most of the novel ideas in the book are folded into this single package. If I had the time, I would build them more gradually into the explanation. As it is, the reader may have to work backwards in the book to explore their construction.

We begin the book by outlining the proposed solution to problems which are described in later sections. The hope is to avoid the appearance of grievance, first presenting the proposal in general terms, before describing many of the reasons for it. The second section of the book, however, is a series of comments on the hidden economics of healthcare. It reflects the author's views after sixty years as a practicing physician in many roles. This section probably reflects most physicians' viewpoint on a number of features of healthcare which the public is seldom exposed to, but many of the details are unfamiliar even to physicians. The importance lies in leading to yet another main proposal, which is to make a deal with the employer community to repair the problems created in the past century of employer-based health insurance. In a sense, employers and unions act as though employer-based insurance is nobody else's business. But because they are heavily funded by tax deduction, nobody owns the concept, and it is fair game for anybody's comment.

The third section contains major working details of Health Savings Accounts, once a fuller theory has been set forth. In particular, investment and constitutional issues are expanded. It could expand on the details and requirements of adjusting employer-based insurance, except that is scarcely necessary, and in any event is beyond my control. I originally saw the employer-based proposal as incidental to Health Savings Accounts, but the employer community could well regard it as the only issue worth talking about.

At the end, a sixth section of this book extracts almost fifty specific legislative proposals which require attention before final Lifetime proposals could be completely operational. Lifetime viewpoints are the ultimate goals; we have too many one-viewpoint silos. The author is reluctantly brought to the conclusion that both employer-based health insurance and Medicare are solutions now outgrowing their former usefulness. Obamacare is regarded as not really a reform, but a nationalization of the finance system, with intended reforms remaining undeclared, just so long as Government decides them. Nobody owns this problem, or its solution. It is a public debate, and a continuing one.

And after all, this is a book, not a political speech. Marketing and administrative costs of HSA will be considerable; all details are expensive, take time to explain. Revenue sources vary, as do sickness costs. Only the HSA concept remains durable throughout, and its basic premise is, you should be in control of your own finances. Therefore, please understand where you might be going. Unfortunately, to do that requires re-examination of a system which served us fairly well for a century, but now causes considerable trouble itself.

Now to jump around, the Supreme Court decision of *King v. Burwell* seems to have assured the Affordable Care Act will be part of our system for some time. However at the same time, health insurance companies have suddenly raised their rates so much it becomes doubtful the nation can afford to continue the ACA approach. Or at least, without abandoning its major role in some other field, like international affairs. Therefore, I discarded any attempt to predict what will happen, and developed an interim plan for making choices.

It was to apply the Health Savings Account approach to everything else except age group 21-66 which apparently will be dominated by

Obamacare until elections settle some issues. Everything else would cover at least as much healthcare cost as the ACA does; but without bipartisanship it would be a stretch to make it work. Adding the two together would considerably increase the savings for mathematical reasons I will explain, and perhaps be the basis for compromise. As I worked through the details however, I decided the thirty million President Obama decided to omit, were better suited to individually tailored solutions, and Medicare was too big to take on as part of a solution. That doesn't seem to leave anybody, but in fact it points straight at children, which I now see have been an invisible stumbling-block, all along. So that's New Health Savings Accounts (N-HSA), plus modified Obamacare, leading to Lifetime (L-HSA) by the back door. Combining two plans that almost work, into one plan that works much better, would be quite an achievement. Meanwhile, we certainly will have an interesting debate. If we could only stir employer-based insurance into the mixture, it might become very exciting, indeed.

George Ross Fisher, MD

Philadelphia

October, 2015

Planning for Prosperity

Health Savings Accounts in Three Variations

Healthcare, A Much Simplified Overview

L et me say at the beginning, what could be repeated in a summary: The present healthcare dilemma has three interlocked parts, scientific, financial, and political. The **scientific component** is capsulized by three symbolic life expectancies: in 1900: age 47, today: age 83, and fifty years from now: age 100. We're living a lot longer, and soon expect the population to divide into thirds (one third getting educated, one third retired, and one third working to support the whole population. It probably won't work very well. Most health reforms amount to finding some way to shift income from the working third to the other two thirds.

The main scientific problem in the past was to avoid dying too young. But the problem in the far future will be living too long, running out of savings. Right now we can imagine having both problems, and few can guess which problem to fear. Maybe there is enough money for one of those two life terminations, but we don't have enough money for both of them, for everyone. We would have to give up something else, like national defense. Let's try to use the same money twice, if we can.

Finance. The payment systems need to be more interchangeable for alternative uses. But be careful. This could seemingly lead to merging Medicare and Social Security (some day) into one interchangeable program. Interchangeability of funds might plausibly seek to be at the family level instead of over-reaching to the level of demographic groups of whole thirds of the population. We do need to devise ways to transfer from one stage of a person's life to another, Saving for a Rainy Day, as it were. Some solutions will inevitably turn into problems. Proposals to integrate all health care into one vertical single-payer medical system would likely clash with more useful integration of Medicare and Social Security. These arguments can possibly wait for a later time, but only if we recognize they remain undecided. Generally speaking, they translate into recognizing that it is easier to shift money than people. Governments regard such shifting with indifference, but we train children from birth to be possessive about their own money. And we elect politicians to see the difference.

Both the insurance <u>spread-the-risk</u> approach and the government <u>pooling</u> process skirt the difficulty there is not enough money to cover both possibilities for everyone. Either to borrow or insure, postpones repayment for a while, that's about all. Meanwhile, healthcare costs are subject to more sudden changes in greater ranges than the economy as a whole.

Finally, let's see if we can put these shifts to work, and get some extra money from investment income, with compound interest working its magic over the whole expanse.

Politics. Meanwhile, we move toward a time when voters who earn money aren't sick, and the sick voters don't earn money. But they all have a vote. Already, we conduct transfers of money on a scale people may rebel against. It must become their own money, in their own accounts, spent later on themselves – rather than forced transfers between demographic groups. At most, we might try extending that to the family unit, and even that should be kept as voluntary as possible..

> *"Constitutional equal justice tends to make political solutions resemble one-size fits all."*

The political issue is central. We wish for equal justice under the law, so political decisions always resemble one-size-fits all. An exaggeration of this is a heedless majority ruling on its own behalf, allowing 51% to have things their way, or the highway. Rights of the minority must be more respected, especially when few can foresee their own future interests. So democracy prizes being slow. Slow, conservative and one-size-fits all. It's hard to know how it came about, but this is the best governing system the world has ever seen, unless one-size fits-all doesn't fit you. Where the solution is to share community resources, even that recourse is unlikely to be satisfactory.

So that's the general nature of our problems. Healthcare does become less expensive in the long run, even though more expensive in the short run. And through recent advances of financial management, Health Savings Accounts can generate surprising amounts of extra money on their own, overall helping with the other problems. The abstruse issue of inflation also arises here, where you might not expect it, because if trillions of dollars eventually migrate into passive investments through Health Savings Accounts, the elderly will hold shareholder voting rights they would be unwilling to surrender. The course of further inflation, the main concern of the elderly, would shift toward the hands of savers, away from borrowers. Unfortunately, what the proper balance is, isn't yet clear.

Employer-Based Health Insurance in a Nutshell

Modern health insurance is a century old in America, and much of its interesting history is irrelevant to present controversies. However, a few features are important to know as a preliminary. It started as a benevolence by business to its employees after the First World War, at a time when most businesses were family-owned. In 1945, Henry J. Kaiser discovered health insurance could mostly be financed by successful corporate employers donating it to their employees, thus transforming a gift of health insurance into a business expense.

The gift soon became accepted as a normal part of wages, so the pay packet drifted downward to expect it. The employer paid the same total tax, but the employee got a tax reduction. When the corporate income tax rate became double the individual rates, the employer got twice the deduction the employee got. As other taxes began to be based on the remaining pay packet rather than the total wage cost, employers escaped the extra tax. The employer overall got more benefit from the tax shelter than the employee did, and he got it for every one of his employees. Less successful businesses (with less tax to pay) often could not share in these last two features, and often preferred to remain with Subchapter S incorporation, although their employees lost out on deductions and in general were the only losers. If this is new to you, read that last paragraph again.

In this way, the tax exemption became a normal part of business life, and tinkering was greatly resented. By a century later, CEOs have turned this matter over to Personnel offices and financial officers, forgetting its complicated mechanics, and have gone on to other matters. It was a gift, so the employees were seldom consulted about its details, and in time most employees became oblivious to them. The situation began to be known as "third-party" insurance, and in time the basic decisions were made without much consideration of either the employer or the employee, who seldom raised a fuss. In the course of a century, it was the wishes of the insurer that mainly dominated the decisions, mostly because decisions had to be made, and nobody else cared very much. A century of unopposed decision-making gradually warped the employer-based system into a very expensive, inexplicably complicated combination of incentives, all leading to escalating prices for healthcare. The foxes were in charge of the hen house, and everybody's incentive was to let healthcare prices drift upward.

It is the organization of incentives rather than greed or malice which led to this predicament, so it is not justified to attack anyone. But someone who has benefits to defend can become quite offended when the benefits are disparaged. For insurance company reasons, the useless and expensive 20% copayment system has persisted, while the deductible has remained too small to serve a purpose. For political count-the-votes reasons, the benefit package has favored numerous small pills over major surgery, warping the reimbursement system in favor of more transactions. As disease has receded in younger people, young people have demanded "something for their money", even though it distorted the benefit package unwisely to use limited funds for small bills rather than large ones. Short-term gains repeatedly triumphed over long-term considerations, slowly but relentlessly warping it away from intended directions.

It is my feeling the average reader needs a little more background: in overfunding for Retirement, buying out Medicare gradually, first and last year-of-life insurance, and the plight of the latecomer to lifetime health insurance – before we are ready to solve problems in the last five sections of this book. There are a few other salient issues to learn, and a century of history to skip, before the casual reader is likely to be ready to address the issues in central contention. So, skip it or study it, that's what the rest of this section is all about.

Health Savings Account in a Nutshell

There are now reported to be 15 million subscribers to Health Savings Accounts, growing at about a million new subscribers a year, with hardly any advertising. It's really a very simple concept, consisting of two parts. The Savings Account is pretty much like any other savings account, and I understand one New York Bank has 700,000 accounts. You are allowed to make deposits up to $3350 a year, terminating when Medicare begins, at age 66. At that point, any balance in the account is turned into an IRA, and may be used for any purpose after paying income tax. When you make withdrawals for other purposes there is a penalty tax of 20%. They may be used for legitimate healthcare purposes, <u>without</u> taxation. The statutory basis for this is that deposits are tax-deductible, and withdrawals for health are tax-sheltered; the rest of the rules are regulation. Most accounts are linked to a debit card for medical purchases.

> *"Two working parts: (1) Tax-exempt saving fund (2) Catastrophic (high deductible) health insurance"*
>
> **HSA in Essence**

In order to make deposits, the subscriber must link the account to a high-deductible health insurance policy. It is often difficult to obtain a public quote on price, which must mean the price is highly competitive and variable. Changes in the environment make for price changes which are almost not worth printing in a pamphlet. Many account managers insist on linking to a specific brokerage account, either subsidiaries, or linked by fee arrangements; such details are to be frowned upon. The new investor should be aware that most index funds of the entire domestic market return slightly less than 12%, but the manager of a fund subtracts overhead and passes on a variable amount to the customer. The amount of this return on investment is critical, and the ability to move accounts to a new manager if dissatisfied is an important feature but an optional one. It is also important for the catastrophic insurer to have made price arrangements with local hospitals which are competitive. A price of one and a quarter times the Medicare rate is on the high end.

Most investment manager are not fiduciaries, they are brokers. That is, they have no legal obligation to put the customer's interest ahead of their own. It is reported that most new subscribers are between the age of 30 and 45. That is, old enough to have some savings, young enough to gather meaningful income before being used. Actuaries report the average yearly cost is about 30% less than conventional health insurance, but price quotes are difficult to get on anything but an individual basis, and there may be some tacit underwriting.

The Deal Breaker

The current "healthcare reform" really concentrates on the payment mechanism for healthcare. It may nurse grander ambitions, but it directly confronts only one of the many problems with healthcare delivery – whether poor people can afford it. Much is made of the electronic medical record but its impact is mostly one of user annoyance. The fundamental structures of hospitals and medical practice, growing out of the much older employer-based system, are pretty much unchanged. The configuration is mainly the employer-based system.

In the far future, control of payments may eventually be used as a hammer to control healthcare, but that goal has never been articulated, and the slow pace of the past six years suggests any such goal is distant, indeed. For practical purposes, the Affordable Care Act (ACA) reduces to a payment mandate – universal health insurance for everyone regardless of cost, subsidizing those whose insurance costs exceed 8% of income. Opponents reply: Since 87% of the people who bought insurance on a Federal Exchange did so with subsidies, the cost could seemingly bankrupt the country, crippling more important priorities. In general, I sympathize with both emotional responses (care for the poor but don't wreck the economy), except for one essential point. In almost every foreign health plan, the government becomes generous with trivial items and stingy with expensive ones. Plenty of cough drops, but not many chest x-rays. Or plenty of chest x-rays, but woefully few MRIs. When you see what others have done, you get a better idea of what we might be facing.

The deal-breaker for me is the kind of insurance selected to be mandatory. Catastrophic (high-deductible) health insurance without frills would be far more suitable, and considerably cheaper. Bare-

> *"The deal-breaker for me, is the type of insurance made mandatory."*

boned catastrophic insurance has both a top limit and a bottom limit, and uses money as an indemnity measure, not elastic definitions like "service" benefits. (Indemnity pays for your cost, not your disease.) Without prior experience, new insurance entrants should not guess at their risks, either individually or collectively. Service benefits might be considered after long and stable experience, but for a beginning new program, they tilt the balance between patient risk and insurer risk entirely too much in favor of patients whose real client could be the elected politician. If everyone is playing fair, there should not be much difference in cost outcome. But the present uproar in Greece and Cyprus demonstrates the risk of the political approach of giving

> *"The higher the deductible, the lower the premium."*
> **High-Deductible Catastrophic Insurance.**

elected officials the keys to your life expectancy. Indeed catastrophic high-deductible insurance may be the only universally acceptable alternative to whatever we now have, but which we criticize so vigorously.

The problem with the Affordable Care Act is not that it excludes too much, but that it scolds too much and improves too little. By utilizing its principle that **the higher the deductible, the lower the premium**, the flexibility of catastrophic coverage could almost rest its case. By adjusting the premium, anyone might afford it; by adjusting the deductible, anything might be a covered service. But the general philosophy we would hope for, is to cover no non-essentials until the last essential service has been covered. The choice of deductible threshold defines the coverage by simultaneously defining the premium, allowing both the paying public and the subsidizing public to bid in the same auction. Deficit financing is much harder to conceal if you play by indemnity rules. Nothing else I know of can make a similar claim. I tend to resist anything with the word "mandatory" in it, but catastrophic health insurance offers a flexibility which might justify an exception.

Of course, flexibility is only valuable if you use it. With its high deductible, **catastrophic coverage** excludes small-cost items. Like birth control pills, I'm sorry to have to say. High-cost coverage automatically means expensive but relatively infrequent health issues, which in present circumstances means inpatient hospital care. Defining low-cost benefits as "service" benefits, usually undermines Catastrophic insurance. It converts the ACA into scarcely more than a collection of small mandatory benefits, all of which defeat the purposes of a high deductible.

The effect of all this is to suggest high-cost items are the enemy, but in fact they are usually the most important benefit to include. Collecting all small benefits into Savings Accounts substitutes patient choice for unlimited bureaucracy, shifting the selection burden to the subscriber and his doctor. High deductibles make them turn to their doctors for advice when they are worried. That's quite different from requiring a slip of paper from a doctor whenever things are expensive.

First and Last Years of Life Health Insurance

Here's an idea which has been bouncing around in my head for several decades. The first year of everybody's life resembles the last year in several unique ways. Everybody has a first and last year of life, but essentially no one pays for his own healthcare during those two years. They are pretty expensive years, amounting to 3% for the birth year and something like twenty percent for the last one, so if these costs were removed from the calculation of health insurance premiums, it would make a substantial relief. So, why don't we invent a kind of health insurance which pays for those two years, relieving the rest of the system of this cost? Paying for it during years of employment, would shift the cost to the earning third, from the non-earning two thirds.

> *"Health care can't get more basic than being born or dying."*
> **Irreducible Minimums.**

This kind of health insurance would have to be retrospective, but the dates alone would make it fairly easy to administer. Someone else would have to pay these costs first, so it's likely this insurance would largely be a new insurance company. It would reimburse another insurance company which could prove it legitimately paid the cost, that the prices were fair, etc. Whether this was a mandatory requirement for people who had this payment responsibility, or a function of the government on everybody's behalf – makes less difference because this health issue is universal, so it might as well be unspecified. On the other hand, if it is made a voluntary liability of people who have payment responsibilities, they would require some proof the whole arrangement is on the up and up.

Insurance executives would seek some way to pay average costs for the whole country, since it would simplify their job not to get into the nitty-gritty of itemized charges. That's what has happened with the Affordable Care Act, and it hasn't proved to be acceptable to all parties.They might have to be satisfied with partial steps in that direction, paying hospital bills only, or institutions only, since arguing over the cost of diapers and baby-sitting might be too contentious. There are, after all, many costs incurred during the first and last years of life which are probably not legitimate health care costs, but under the circumstances would naturally have a sort of medical flavor to them. It thus would seem like a good beginning to have the people who are interested in one side of the business or the other, get together and construct a joint proposal which they consider workable. The people who are likely to be presented with the bill would have slightly different viewpoints, and several proposals might result.

This idea, in somewhat greater detail, might be examined in conjunction with universal Catastrophic health insurance. There would be many overlaps, and practicality might dictate the choice. But when we seem to have got it about right, either one of these choices or possibly some hybrid of both, would likely be a better thing to make into mandatory coverage. Or at least mandatory in the sense it might become illegal to have coverage for less universal, and less urgent coverage – unless you have one of these more basic coverages, first. Society, whatever it may claim, has almost always proved to be pretty stingy. So, other coverages would have to be depended on to provide the extras, and to defend their practicality as insurance. It would seem to be a useful thing, to have one insurer arguing cost, and the other insurance company arguing quality, so that neither one would try to threaten the other with unbearable legal costs as the main pressure.

Overfunding for Retirement

Independence Blue Cross (of Philadelphia) has imaginatively designed a Health Savings Account product for retirement purposes, by allowing the employer or the employee to overfund an HSA with $750 annual contributions, looking ahead to the employee's retirement. The HSA part is presented as an add-on to conventional Blue Cross, although it is unclear whether that is required. Independence Blue Cross should be given credit for a good idea. Whether it supplements health insurance before retirement, is apparently left up to the employee, but of course it does supplement any other after-retirement arrangements the employee may have, because the HSA continues on after Blue Cross itself terminates at age 66.

Since employers may soon face an un-suspended requirement to provide health insurance meeting ACA requirements, the high deductible from the government plan might simultaneously supply the high-deductible requirement for the HSA. This seems an efficient way to address present uncertainties, and could provide the basis for compromise discussions between the two political parties on the whole subject of fringe benefits. High-deductible is good; adding subsidies confuses the intent. Keep them separate.

Overfunding is always a good idea for subscribers to HSA, whatever their other program features. Politicians avoid overfunding anything because of voter reaction, so private plans are generally more flexible than public ones, while voters tend to complain that instead of overfunding, taxes should be reduced. The program is so new, and its time periods so distant, that unintentional gaps in coverage are always possible. If worries prove unfounded, overfunding leads to more money for retirement, hardly a tragedy.

> **Over-investment in Health Savings Accounts – The Retirement Alternative.** Because it's a new program, with financing uncertainties, we advise everyone with an HSA to consider **overfunding** it as a precaution. Just about everyone could readily use surpluses for some of his retirement. Although the employer only donates $750 per year, the law allows a total of $3350 as a maximum, and so a $2600 personal supplement is required in the following three hypothetical but typical situations. At this level, the employer contribution is a small factor; what really matter are inflation, and interest return. And starting at an early age.

Example One. Let's say an employee starts the program at age 21 and remains with the company until retiring at age 66, contributing $3350 per year to the HSA (in the Blue Cross plan, $750 comes from the employer, and the employee must supplement $2600 from personal funds). (It makes no difference whether the employee rises through promotions or remains at entry level; the maximum is the same.) Result: the employee receives a taxable retirement income at age 66 from the HSA to IRA transfer of $81,616 per year until age 83, dropping to 66,642 with 3% inflation. If life expectancy of 93 is anticipated, the yearly annuity drops to $65,621, dropping to 48,595 with inflation.

Example Two. Another employee enrolls at age 21 but retires to get married at age 26. At age 66, until death, there is a yearly $23,423 retirement income assuming life expectancy of 83, and dropping to

19,125 with 3% inflation. Assuming 93, the annuity is $ 18,832 with and $ 13,946 without 3% inflation.

Example Three. An employee joins the firm at age 61 and remains until age 66. His retirement income is $1,886 per year, dropping to $ 1,540 with inflation, Assuming expectancy of 93, he gets $1,516 yearly, or $1,123 after 3% inflation.

In the examples, many things jump out. The first is the large disparity between what five years of work will get you, starting at age 21, compared with the almost pitiful amount a person age 61 will get for the same absolute, and maximum allowable, contribution. The difference between examples is the difference between whole social classes. That difference of course is made up out of the income compounded internally for 40 years. And the moral is clear, a small steady investment at an early age is worth far more than the same investment at the end of a working life. It happens to cost the employer the same, either way, and he may not realize it. His viewpoint will depend on what value he places on maturity and experience in an older employee, as compared with vigor and strength in a younger one; the pension costs would be the same.

However, this is a major change in pension design, and people should familiarize themselves with it. The employer can make far more difference in an employee's life with the selection of savings plan, than with salary. Perhaps another way of looking at it is the employee gets to keep the interest compounding in an HSA, whereas in other plans the employer gets to keep it. Or, depending on how the contract is written, some middle-man gets to keep it. The old defined benefit plans placed much more emphasis on training and experience, and much less on the age and duration of enrollment. It's a new ball game. For example, there is no reason why an employer couldn't have two plans, with an optional choice, one for young people, the other for late comers.

The second point revolves around the interest rate being paid. The investment manager, whether in-house or by way of a vendor, is able to earn, and should be able to earn, 12% on an index fund of the common stock of the whole American market. Inflation at a steady rate of 3% for a century, reduces that return to 9%, net of inflation. How much is the employee entitled to?

Much depends on whether inflation is pre-deducted in advance, or calculated at some later time. If an employee is paid less than 3% per year for his HSA, he actually loses money on the exchange. If he is paid 7.5% gross, he only receives 4% net of inflation, in spite of surrendering half of the net gain (4.5% of 9%) to the broker or manager.

In this example we have arbitrarily assigned him 6.5%, which is 3.5% net of inflation, yielding well over half of the margin to the broker. I have to wonder whether the services provided are really worth more than 1% (for example, one nearby trillion dollar firm only charges a tenth as much), so it seems as though a fair return to the investor/subscriber should be 5%, net of inflation, net of fees, or 8% gross. So, be careful to identify whether inflation is anticipated, or only calculated after it happens. Sometimes, both approaches are adopted, and someone is seriously affected by not noticing it.

That means the price debate ranges between 3% (no profit to the investor at all) and 8% (essentially the wholesale price). Throughout this book, I have generally adopted 6.5% as an average, mainly to be safely conservative and avoid arguments. The marketplace will eventually settle on the "right" price, but if it's less than 3.5% net of inflation, it's less than a quarter of the wholesale price. Eventually, I expect the price to be knocked up to 8%, net of inflation, or 11% gross. The ultimate effect of this price pressure on the cost of health care, would be considerable, indeed. Sustainable retirement would come into sight, and as we have mentioned, the price of healthcare is linked to it.

Now, I don't want to be accused of starting a revolution, but my calculator tells me if passive investment could achieve 6.5% income return, the first of the three examples cited above would receive a retirement income of $81,616 per year. And the old fellow who decided to work for a few years to build up his retirement, would receive $1,866. The youngster who worked five years and then quit, could look forward to a pension of $23,423 per year. Something tells me this is too destabilizing, so I'm not going to get impaled on the barricades discussing it. Ultimately, it probably reflects a reduction of transactional costs by electronics, which has not yet worked its way through to retail consumers. So, one way or another, something is going to happen, and it's up to all of us to make sure it is benevolent.

Overfunding health insurance by one means or another is a very good idea if you can afford it – and you keep your wits about you.

Buying-Out Medicare

O n his 66th birthday, a Health Savings Account owner has only one choice: to turn any surplus from healthcare into an IRA (Individual Retirement Account), for taxable retirement living. However, that's a step better than Medicare or employer-based insurance alone, which return the unused surplus to the <u>donor</u> of the gift, either the government or the employer, in the form of reduced premium cost. However, economists agree the salary soon adjusts downward to treat the confidently expected gift as part of wage costs. Therefore, the health insurance is more expensive than it would be if the surplus were returned to the beneficiary. These forms of health insurance have been dominant so long, everyone feels they describe necessary features of health insurance, rather than simply terms of a contract negotiated by parties other than the beneficiary.

The presumption is made the individual has Medicare, so any accumulated surplus in his HSA needs to be spent after age 66, but not on health, since he assumes he will then be completely covered. This presumption is strengthened when the employees of a group plan are merged into a group, so any surplus is an average of the group, not specific to the individual. Data is not available to determine whether the size of this issue is enough to worry about. But a pathway probably was not created for overfunding Medicare to create retirement savings through employer-based insurance. In the first place, surplus does not exist. In the second place, any surplus was probably expected to flow back into Medicare to reduce its cost. In 1965, it was probably expected that Social Security would fill this need, but increasing longevity has created resistance to enhancing all entitlement programs.

However, if changes in laws and regulations would make it possible, there might be other choices, one of which would be to overfund Medicare coverage, continue the HSA, and spend the generated

20

surplus on retirement. But notice this: as things stand, if you don't need Medicare any more, you don't get anything back and the government can spend the surplus on battleships. Just as, in plain fact, a commercial insurance company can spend a surplus on executive salaries. It's not fair to say Medicare will "never" have a surplus. By design, any surplus will always be used for healthcare, because that's thought to be part of "share the risk". It's a design feature common in share the risk programs, although not a devastating one.

In short, the designers of Medicare never imagined it would run a surplus, and at present it is far from it. But in the long, long run, scientists will eventually cure those chronic diseases of the elderly, and then there might actually be such a surplus. It is already clear things are moving in the direction of making Social Security a larger if not more important program than Medicare – in the short run – and could largely replace Medicare, in the long run. Because expensive illness is often fatal illness, a great many people do not survive it. So, one ray of hope in this situation is relatively few people will have both devastations, so the future is probably one expensive entitlement transforming into the other with relatively little overlap. In that case, dual catastrophes are best addressed by insurance. With luck, the people who drop dead without warning or cost will equal the number of overlaps, smoothing down national expense to only two groups, which eventually merge into one as science merges chronic disease into the growing group whose problem is outliving their savings. There are other ways of approaching that problem, but at least a flexible health program could provide a source of funding for it, and a general outline of where it might be headed. Notice that compound interest works in favor of this solution, and could be an important component. In fact, unknown treatments will increase future expense, but by definition are not counted. Therefore, statistical projections can show a revenue surplus after the age of 90, which may in fact never materialize.

Therefore it would be easier to pass a seemingly meaningless amendment, right now, while it doesn't cost anything. We've just shown how HSA does it, and Medicare could do it too, if it tried. The more likely circumstance would be to get a reduction of either payroll deductions or Medicare premiums in return for surrendering some particular benefit, like transfusions for members of Jehovah's Witnesses. At the moment, religious objectors cause lawsuits and other commotion, just because they don't want some particular feature of health insurance, and actually I can think of no reason why we should make it mandatory. In fact, doing things for someone's own good is a suspect idea, generally.

The long-range reasoning, however, is this: in 2015 the great need is for flexibility. Some of us will need to spend every dime we have on staying alive. And some of us will need to save every dime we can, in order not to outlive our retirement funds. But that probably won't be the same dilemma, fifty years from now. Almost every one of us could be threatened with poverty during extended retirement into an undefinable longevity. It strains the imagination to think of ways to pay for both the present elaborate Medicare <u>and</u> an extended retirement in addition. So, by that time, I fully expect people to have come to the realization that Medicare must be liquidated piece by piece. Not to fund Obamacare, but to pay for their own retirement. When you go to a funeral every week, the idea doesn't usually occur that dying too early might ever become a thing of the past.

> *"Neither employer-based nor Medicare, returns unused surplus to subscribers."*

For one thing, I expect "rent-seeking" to soak up a lot of the savings from people not getting quite so sick. Rent-seeking will take many forms, like Botox injections and cosmetic surgery. Or like elaborate hospital equipment and excessive salaries, or like too much stand-by but essentially unused equipment. It may sometimes be hard to tell where the money is going, but costs will surely fail to fall as rapidly as illness can disappear. We will need a way for people to perceive this, and for them voluntarily to start saving for it by gradually opting out of Medicare. It won't be an all-or-none issue; people will perceive it at different rates. Therefore, we need to provide a way to get out of Medicare in steps, and individually one by one, over a period of decades. For political reasons, the use of a surplus should be limited to your own retirement living. All of this is called "planning ahead".

Proposal 1: At present, Health Savings Accounts are limited to age 21-66. There should be no age limits at either end, and some provision should be made for inheritance of surplus to newborn children, sufficient to cover their healthcare up to age 21. (3320)

Proposal 2: At present, contributions to Health Savings accounts are limited to $3500 per year, age 21 to 66. This should be changed to an aggregate lifetime amount, at least until latecomers have had an adequate transition to the program. (3320)

Health Savings Accounts provide the flexibility to do this, but at present many Medicare program details are awkwardly designed to anticipate the need. Right now, the program is not sufficiently modular to permit dropping one feature but retaining others, and letting the funds follow the needs. And designing partial proposals is inhibited by political terror that the public will misinterpret motives. So the first step is for people like me, who have nothing to lose, to step forward and start talking about it. The need for retirement money is looming ahead; we need to prepare Medicare for gradual liquidizing, to pay for it.

The first step is probably to design a way to buy out of Medicare, save some money by substituting an HSA for their healthcare, and buy something more appealing with the surplus. The first version will probably be crude and awkward, but it provides a platform to build on. Most politicians, whatever they may think of Medicare and its financing, regard talk of privatizing Medicare as political suicide, so we should be thinking of pilot studies, think tanks, and experimental projects. The old folks who have, or will soon have, Medicare coverage regard it as such a treasure, they tell their elected representatives that privatizing Medicare is the third rail of politics: touch it and you are dead. But a Washington sage once remarked that if things can't go on, they will stop. So, what would it require, to induce potential Medicare beneficiaries to select something else, before circumstances abruptly force it on them?

That's probably not the best way to go about it. The early initiatives should be generated by scientific advances. The likelihood is great that science will cure one or two of the big five (cancer, diabetes, Parkinsonism, Alzheimer's Disease, schizophrenia) and bit by bit, Medicare will get cheaper in spite of the rent-seeking. As it does, it will seem attractive to increasing numbers of people, to consider cheaper health insurance, shifting Medicare funding to retirement income. The rules should be relaxed to let early-adopters test the changing environment. We already have a flexible funding vehicle in Health Savings Accounts, and fifteen million existing subscribers who will endorse it.

The Problem With Medicare. Medicare is 50% self-funded by payroll deductions and premiums, and is 50% subsidized by the federal government. The old folks get a dollar for fifty cents, and are not about to give it up. They obviously should get their own fifty cents back. It's the fifty cents of government subsidy which is at issue, and the published budget should reflect that fact. Just notice how retirees display almost no interest in the Obamacare controversy, except for one thing. Old folks are uneasy that funding for Medicare might get squeezed in order to finance Obamacare, particularly if the two were in the same budget compartment. When the conversation gets around to that point, retirees suddenly wake up and start talking loudly. If the discussion centered on the subsidy, things might subside, somewhat.

Medicare Buyout

Item *	Subscriber	Government
$84,000 from H.S.A.	(-)	(+)
$42,00 Payroll Deduction	(+)	(-)
$42,000 Medicare Premium	(+)	(-)
$26,000 Tax Reductions	(+)	(-)
$82,000 Foreign Debt	0	(+)
	$200,000.00	$60,000

* Rough Figures for Differing Ages

But hold on. A retiree approaching his 66th birthday has already pre-paid approximately a quarter of the costs of Medicare, and when he joins, his premiums will later amount to another quarter of the cost. That 50% is the retiree's share of the present costs of Medicare, and naturally he doesn't expect to see it disappear. The 50% subsidy provided by the government, on the other hand, is what concerns everyone. Even the people who advocate "single payer" systems are talking about extending Medicare to the whole population, gradually perhaps, but probably including the 50% subsidy to everyone. Since healthcare now consumes 18% of Gross Domestic Product, are we willing to see 9% of GDP go from the private sector to the public sector in extra taxes? Or in increased borrowing from foreign nations? We will have to let the politicians wrestle with issues like that, but it will be hard to persuade the public to go along with it.

Meanwhile, let's see what persuasion can do, if we offer a good enough deal. For a start, let's presume someone in his late fifties had invested in his HSA while he was young, and is approaching the age where he could augment his retirement income from a substantial balance in his IRA (recently converted from HSA). Then, let us say he also wakes up to the realization he gets a second tax deduction from an HSA if he spends extra retirement money on medical care, either on Medicare payroll deductions or Medicare premiums. And if he stops spending some other obligation, he effectively gets a further tax deduction from spending the money on something else which is tax-free. Potentially, that could add a few thousand dollars a year to his income from age 21 to the day he dies. It's a very attractive goal, and while it really would be legitimately spent on healthcare, Congress might well decide they can't afford to lose that much tax revenue.

So, the rumination goes, the proposal must somehow save some money for the Government, too. If the subscriber were allowed to make a deal to buy out his Medicare, he might make a payment out of his HSA of about $86,000 untaxed, which with 6.5% declining income, would repay the costs of Medicare throughout his remaining life expectancy, all from the invested lump sum. That might seem like enough on paper, but the government has been going in debt for some time to foreigners, and would like to stop doing that. If possible, it would like to pay back the earlier loans. If you include this debt, the Medicare cost is revealed as greater than it seems. Furthermore, the GAO will quickly tell you, if you save tax money, you unfortunately make it harder to balance the federal budget. The details of all this may be hard to explain, but the general sense of it all, is pretty clear.

Let's qualify the simplifications. Different people will have different payroll deductions, at different ages. To some extent, these balance out, because if you have a larger balance in your HSA, you are likely to be older, and likely to have paid more into your Medicare payroll deductions. And to some extent, averages will cancel out and vary with the economy from time to time. A change in the tax code would scramble all of these numbers, but it's preliminary. Medicare is best privatized in pieces, and for that you need prices, so a preliminary pricing should be devised for those people who for religious or other reasons, would be interested. Furthermore, accumulating money of this order will require normal interest rates, not abnormally low ones as at present. Since that time is hard to predict, it is necessary to supply minimum interest guarantees, best approximated by index funds of 10-year treasury bonds. Buying out Medicare is a very delicate matter, and should be approached very slowly. The first step is to talk about it without starting a panic. The initial appeal will be found among those who perceive a greater risk from outliving their income than their risk of a major illness cost. They are rare at present, but times will change.

The Plight of the Latecomer to HSA

M edicare had been in existence for fifteen years when Health Savings Accounts were designed. Medicare was popular and apparently permanent. Accordingly, the HSA proposal was intended to phase out when the individual became a Medicare recipient. Since there might be an unspent surplus at that time, it was provided that the surplus be turned into an IRA, partly as a gesture of deference to Senator William Roth of Delaware, who was the originator of the tax-exempt fund idea. The consequence is that the HSA now bridges the transition, between health care and prolonged longevity. That's a feature now seen to be an enhancement.

However, experience with the program shows we overlooked something. The plans are attracting a following between the ages of 35 and 50, which is to say they turn unattractive to people 50 to 66, who ought to be in their highest years of earning. On interviewing them, the difficulty seems to be that diseases start increasing at about that age, and a depletion of the account gives it scant opportunity to recover before the program terminates. Compound interest is fine, but if you have used it up for disease A, it cannot compound enough to support disease B. By contrast, a subscriber at age 35 might well be in a position to pay for one bout of illness, followed by compound interest build-up. So the plan covered two or three more severe illnesses before age 66 is attained. The contribution limit of $3300 annually is just not enough to provide a comfortable margin. Furthermore, the purpose of the limit is not clear. If a subscriber contributes more, it would be his own money, not the government's. True, it would be tax exempt, but a very large proportion of the population are tax-exempt through their employer, anyway. People whose income is concentrated may be especially affected, such as those who sell a farm or business, or athletes. Finally, everything said about unexpected illness would be true of unexpected stock market fluctuations.

> **Proposal 3:** The annual limit of deposits to HSA should be increased by a COLA based on medical costs, rather than the cost of living. Furthermore, the limit should be a lifetime limit rather than an annual one. At present, this would substitute a lifetime limit of $132,000 for an annual limit of $3300.

This proposal, while welcome, may still not be enough. The employee with recent experience with healthcare costs, has by the age of 50 come to realize that the personal cost of an HSA has three sources: the deposits which we have mentioned; plus the premium of his required Catastrophic insurance; plus the compound interest rate which his HSA manager is allowing to pass through to him. Additional deposits cost the manager nothing, but the insurance premium and the interest rate are passed through to him from vendors, and their cost is largely obscure to the customer. "Kickbacks" are particularly obscure.

First, the interest rate. The stock market has gone up 12% a year for a century. With transaction costs of perhaps 0.5%, the customer should also subtract 3% for inflation. That creates the remote possibility of paying 8.5% to the customer, and we have in this book generally assumed a net return of 6.5%, with a profit to the middle-men of 2.0%, assuming the middle-man accepts the risk of "black swan" volatility. This is generally about 50% every 28 years. However, the broker probably does not look at it that way. He notices the stock market has gone down in the past few months, may go down more in the next year, and might then take ten of fifteen years to recover to a profitable level. Furthermore, new HSA subscribers may well be young and improvident, have few assets to supply a cushion, and a background of judging a consultant's value by the labor he applies, rather than the risks he takes. The customer wants 6.5%, the broker offers 1%. Each sincerely believes the other is cheating him.

Perhaps a simpler way to summarize the unfortunate confrontation is to recognize it is going to be difficult to support 6.5% retail interest rates in an environment of 1% bank rates, and historically low interest rates, generally. That is particularly true in an environment of falling stock market prices. Unless it can be convincingly shown that someone in this circle is making outrageous profits, or unless someone is willing to put up the capital to buy this business at a discount, the following dangers must be faced and surmounted:

1. The medical customer will eventually resort to what he did in the 1930's. He will neglect his teeth, his gallstones, his varicose veins and hemorrhoids, his eyeglass refractions, and other optional, delayable, services. Consequently, the accident rooms of hospitals will be full of treatable but neglected cases.

2. The stockbrokers will recognize that the era of $250 commissions is over, and the retail customer is going to buy index funds over the Internet from wholesalers, and conduct his medical business dealings out of a bank safe deposit box. The history of discounts in closed-end investment funds, is part of this conversation.

3. The insurance companies will surrender their surveillance role, and strip down to a re-insurance role. Something like the PSRO (Professional Standards Review Organization, see Senator Wallace Bennett of Utah) will take their place.

4. The hospitals can survive a long time on their present surplus assets, particularly buildings. In time, much of their role will be taken over by retirement villages. Doctors and pharmaceutical companies will be squeezed in ways unique to maintaining their function, more or less.

Which will we choose, if we are headed toward a 1930s depression? All of them. But assuming for the moment that things aren't so bad, let's start with #2. The stockbrokers are doomed, anyway. Almost all banks have some empty floor space, where a fee-only wealth advisor can function with his computer terminal. Alternatively, CPAs can absorb a new business model, in addition to filling out tax forms. One thing is not going to remain the same: the finance industry has a whole lot of disintermediation to do.

Classical Health Saving Accounts (C-HSA): In Summary

I t's only a beginning, but the reader now has a summary of where the Classical Health Savings Account stands, with a few suggested amendments to make it better. Remember, with essentially no changes and with minimal marketing effort, C-HSA has acquired fifteen or so million subscribers. Certain features need to be emphasized before it can extend to the rest of life, and harmless modifications made to accommodate the extensions. At the moment, the appeal is mostly to people between the ages of thirty and fifty, while with a few additions it could extend to everyone who wants it. Beyond that, it stumbled onto some features which would make an excellent foundation for wealth creation, for those who don't believe everyone should just invent something and become a billionaire. But to achieve it we have to get past the idea that everything in the public sector must disappear into a black hole, never to return to private hands. Read on, but handle with care.

> **"FLEXIBILITY:**
> *Health Insurance,*
> *plus Retirement*
> *Income if you*
> *survive."*

Hidden Advantages, Mostly Unexploited. C-HSA has the flexibility to manage the transition between health insurance and retirement income. Health insurance is the primary need of the past, retirement income the primary need of the future. It's a lucky feature that relatively few people have both problems, because very few of us could afford to address both of them. At one time, health care was a major concern of employees; nowadays, it is a major concern of retirees. The day will eventually come when so few get seriously ill, other than terminal care, that we can <u>fund retirees for retirement living, and let them dip into the savings if they occasionally get sick</u>. But that's at least a generation away. At every stage, there must be some who generate a surplus, because otherwise some will remain impoverished.

The C-HSA lets you judge your own needs as they come up, rationing what you think you need less of, in order to pay for what you suppose is your likely future need. That's the 2015 problem, and it has no good solution except flexibility – and good luck. Because of the fruits of research, the 2050 problem is going to be retirement income, and it will need a source of revenue. The flexibility of C-HSA allows this choice to be made individually, and eventually permits Medicare to be liquidated to finance it. C-HSA scarcely needs any changing to make this adjustment; Medicare is the program which needs to face the future, make itself modular, and provide ways for people to buy their way out of it, in pieces. Until changes are made to invite partial buy-outs, there is little HSA can do except buy out of Medicare entirely. It will be a long time before many people will take such a big step, but much sooner, they will surely see parts of it they would like to drop in favor of – flexibility.

> **"BOUNDARIES**: *Any surplus belongs to the subscriber."*

Substantial Improvements, Without Disturbing the Basic Structure. Much will depend on the early administration of the Affordable Care Act. If it cannot accommodate the needs of big business in their suspended negotiations, or if it proves to be inordinately expensive, it will collapse. Most of the many Republican candidates for President have endorsed HSA as a substitute policy, and Mrs. Clinton has yet to reveal how she will get out of her HMO proposal of ten years ago. By this time, she surely has learned how distasteful the American public finds HMO, when run by non-physicians. In coming chapters we will describe how essentially the same idea was earlier proposed by physicians, and blocked by the Maricopa Decision of a minority of the United States Supreme Court. Physicians never dreamed anyone would direct a medical organization, except physicians, so there is room for revised opinions; but the twists and turns of politics will eventually dictate where physicians will stand. It is amazing how many people want to run medical care, but how few of them want to go to medical school.

The present stance of HSA proposals is that the Affordable Care Act would be improved by substituting Catastrophic health insurance, or else First and Last Years of Life Insurance, for the present hodge-podge collection small mandatory benefits.

> *"Once we all have basics, we can look around for luxuries.*
> **Benefit Package**

The alternatives, either the employer-based system, or the European single-payer system, similarly become unaffordable when made universal. Universal coverage is indeed desirable, but not to the point of defining that nothing is permitted unless it is universal. If we must have mandatory health insurance,

> "WEALTH CREATION:
> *Tax Exemption, Compound Interest, then Passive Investing."*
> **Future Dream**

let it cover basics alone – either universal experiences like birth and death, or universal fears, like massive expense. Any degree of choice by politicians or bureaucrats is intolerable, and choice by physicians is barely tolerable. Once we all have basics, we can look around for luxuries. Is that too much to ask?

The Golden Surprise. In this book, once we have explored some of the Hidden Economics of Healthcare, we will be ready for the big surprise, which is how much money can be created by changing the insurance design. It might take us a decade to perfect, and several chapters to describe. When lifetime coverage seemed to become possible through the pathway of the tax-exempt Savings Account, supported by Catastrophic fail-safe coverage, we made an amazing discovery. As one of the creators of the idea, I can tell you we had no idea the invested income in these accounts could generate so much money.

That came about by our determinedly avoiding government control, and seeking new pathways the government could not follow. It may be a delusion on my part, but I believe the temper of the public will never tolerate government ownership of private business. Although some far Eastern nations have tried it, their present direction is away from it. Even the Indian subcontinent and the more socialist members of the European Union have found it doesn't work. Very few American college students, however liberal, persist in the notion of government

31

running business, once they emerge from the campus into the real world. The African and South American dictatorships wallow in failures of the oligarchy approach, even when supported by economies based on natural resource discoveries. Consequently, I believe we will emerge from this and future recessions with the cultural belief that collective government ownership of the means of production, is a bad idea. I believe wide-spread distribution of common stock will make us stronger capitalists, not weaker ones. That's a hint of what follows.

SECTION TWO

HIDDEN ECONOMICS OF HEALTHCARE

Here are samplings of the reasons Healthcare Reform still isn't going anywhere.

We started this book with high cost as the main driver of public concern about healthcare. Our proposed alternative is the Health Savings Account. However, a central disappointment in the Affordable Care Act grows out of neglecting almost everything the matter with the system, besides cost, especially the cost to poor people. Many problems cannot be cured by spending more tax money, directly or indirectly, and they deserve some time in the debate. We therefore pause to review a number of other issues which are perhaps less obvious, but not necessarily less serious. Chief among them is the employer-based system, which once served us well, but is wearing out its welcome.

The same might be said of Medicare, but that topic is treated later in the book.

Hidden Economics of Healthcare

By this time, the reader has got part of the idea behind writing this book. The Health Savings Account is legal and popular. Because of the difficulties of the Affordable Care Act, I expanded HSA to compete with President Obama's system. The proposed replacement will be described, after we discuss the problems it hopes to repair. Meanwhile, right now there's the Classical Health Savings Account, for those who would like to join the millions of subscribers who already have one.

There's a lot more to suggest, but it must be preceded by some background, mostly about the Employer-based system. It's what our predominant health system has been for a century. It served us well, but may have out-lived its usefulness. We'll return to the expanded Health Savings Accounts (L-HSA) after we bring the reader up to speed about the things underneath it. Leading to a short but rather sweeping proposal for what to do about it.

Employer Based Health Insurance

In 1965, the most fundamental of economic fundamentals reversed itself. America's international trade balance shifted from positive to negative, has remained negative ever since. It's irrelevant that international currency shifted backward to soften the blow; that's what floating currencies are supposed to do. The era of effortless and largely unchallenged American post-war world supremacy was over. From now on, it was to be every one for himself, in Medicine as in every other trade.

A new triumvirate, consisting of hospitals, health insurance, and medical schools asserted medical leadership, fought against each other for domination, and consequently found themselves a prized destination for opportunists. The new name of the game was to gain control of the payment system, and through it control of hospitals, and through them control of the doctors. But the sponsors of the earlier system, the employer-based one, were still around, and to a large extent, still dominate. No proposal for running healthcare could omit physicians from the center of control. Most who attempt it, seek to use medical schools as a surrogate for the practicing profession. However, medical schools are in competition with their alumni by owning hospitals, and the rest of the profession see medical school control as favoring a competitor. They resist it bitterly.

Meanwhile, the doctors had experienced an entirely different socialization by going away to various wars, and discovering how little they needed hospitals. As shown in episodes of the TV series *Mash*, new bonds were formed between a medical band of brothers, operating successfully in tents, not medical centers. This experience comes and goes, but unfortunately there has been such a succession of wars, the experience gets reinforced. One of the great paradoxes of the present medical upheaval is to see government and insurance doing their best to herd doctors back into hospitals so they can be controlled by salaries, rather than by their patients. And while they seem to have largely succeeded, the ACA ambition to control medical care by control of the payment system is appreciably undermined at its interface between institution and profession. It is always an uphill battle, to defend a more expensive, less satisfying, approach; eventually, it is a losing approach. The oppressive cost of everything, the collision between recessions and inflations, seemed to be keeping everybody under control for the time being. But it would be unwise to assume calm will prevail forever, or that a command-and-control arrangement would continue to work through the hospital, without fragmenting somewhere. In a larger sense, a lot of this history was irrelevant. The people really causing commotion were business leaders with an entirely different agenda; their model was Henry J. Kaiser.

Much of the resulting endgame depends on what Washington will be willing to do. Congress will have its own ideas, but Congress is often in a hurry. What isn't complicated, is often politically difficult, and it helps things along if the public has thought about them first. The Supreme Court gives itself more leisure to think, but sometimes that isn't a pure advantage. The President has more staff, but he can't always control it. Medical cost-cutting turns out to be like closing military bases; it has to be gradual, it has to be spread wide and thin, but it must show early benefits quickly. In its first six years, for example, a lot of people must see some benefit, and very few must see their jobs destroyed. All this can be done, but it can't be done repeatedly. The country cannot afford to keep using up its reserves with noble experiments. World affairs and world economics surely present enough distractions, without inventing artificial ones.

On medical affairs, Congress should learn to listen more to doctors and less to our ancillaries. But for this to happen, doctors will have to become more open about their experiences, rather than electing more doctors to Congress, where they become seen as competitors rather than experts. When Congress finally wakes up to the full dimension of what has happened, everybody is going to need some friends he can trust.

In the final section of this book, we will talk a little about some of the thorny transition problems to be expected. It's not a comprehensive discussion, but a wake-up to the healthcare industry and to Congress, about the complexity of some of the implementation problems they are abandoning to the Executive Branch – at everyone's peril.

So, come along, let's learn a few hidden things. Start with employer-based health insurance. That's what we had for the past century, but hardly noticed it. It even helps to know a little of its history.

A Short History of Employer-based Health Insurance. Instead of starting with Bismarck or some other link to a non-American, let's say health insurance in America began as a proposal of Teddy Roosevelt's during the Progressive Era just before the First World War, a century ago. The American Medical Association had a flirtation with Teddy's national health insurance, but came to prefer something like the business community's Blue Cross system, as it eventually

> *"American health insurance traces back to President Teddy Roosevelt"*

evolved during the 1920's. Business scarcely recognized it, but large American companies were beginning to shift control from founding families to stock holders, an evolution which advanced during the next three decades, as a way to extract capital gains taxes to float war debts. To a certain degree, growing shareholder control was a step toward meritocracy; in a human relations sense, it may have been a step backward. The shift extends to only about half of corporations even today. But health insurance and stockholder control of the big companies advanced side by side, scarcely realizing how diminished employer benevolence was undermining the process. We glorified the decline of a semi-feudal system, but we lost something in the process.

It makes a huge difference whether the boss is a paternalistic owner, or the manager of someone else's company. In the first instance he spends his own money, in the other instance his only absolute mandate is to generate money for the stockholders. That's a measurement applied to every "good" manager. Plenty of owners were tight-fisted, and plenty of managers were benevolent. Even today, small businesses (less than a billion dollars in assets) are mostly "Subchapter S" corporations, and about 15% of really large "Subchapter C" corporations are still dominated by founding families. But in spite of frenzied rhetoric about the "rich owner", the shift in attitudes is clear; as founding generations move away from active involvement in their companies, they become less involved with employees. They themselves become more like their hired managers. Current investment trends, moving into index fund passive investing, further widen the distance between stockholders and owners-by-inheritance. The "silo effect" of specialized departments further isolates the core business from non-revenue support departments.

Cost-shifting was an early development, transferred from the business to the hospital. The concept originally underlying Blue Cross was that private rooms should produce enough profit for the hospital to support the poor folks in open wards, whereas semi-private rooms just break even. At first, only a handful of ministers and school teachers were in the semi-private category. When hospital finances improved, more working-class people moved into the semi-private category, the wards shrank in size, and semi-private – became the standard clause in employee contracts. For two hundred years, multi-bed open wards were standard, but semi-private became standard in a single decade. Semi-private nevertheless acquired a charity flavor. The "Blue Cross discount" began to apply to semi-private beds, at the same time semi-private became readjusted to become "standard size" for "service benefits". That is, most employees of corporations started to be cared for at less than actual cost, at the Blue Cross discount-to-business rate, because their contract called for being provided certain services, no matter what they cost. In fact, what they appeared to cost was so distorted by cost-shifting, you couldn't tell who was subsidized. It would not take long for a new standard to be demanded: sharing a room with strangers was so low-class. Private rooms were going to be the only decent thing. Spending other people's money is fun.

And because Blue Cross organizations became dominant during the second World War, their competitors in cash benefits ("indemnity carriers") greatly resented paying more dollars for the same semi-private than Blue Cross patients did. Some of this was doubtless a response to wage and price controls during World War II, a way of raising wages without expanding the (taxable) "pay packet". The response of commercial indemnity carriers was to price their premiums on "experience rating", which especially cut into the profit margin of Blue Cross private-bed patients. The way that worked was, the insurer waited a year to see what inflation had done, and made a trailing readjustment in the following year's premium. One unexpected outcome of this price warfare was to make the hospital reluctant to reveal its tentative charges, wheras the employer demanded to be shown the actual costs of his employees, as well as prices to everybody else. When Blue Cross coverage reached government employees, a new power center gained possession of itemized hospital bills. A new employee representative could easily see how much or how little the government was actually subsidizing charity care. Naturally, as the new source of a benevolence, they claimed they were paying too much.

When Group practices, or HMOs, started to pay for healthcare, they too demanded to see comparable bills, or at least standardized prices. And so it went, with each new wrinkle in payment. Some people paid listed prices, but big groups could afford to send auditors to look at the books. There had long been a three-tier price list, and now there was a six-tier one because of having list prices and actual payments on each of three levels. Soon it began to seem there might be sixty prices for the same thing. Like a stag cornered by barking dogs, the hospital fended off the payers as best it could. Because of the long period of catch-up following the Great Depression and then the Second World War, hospitals usually needed new buildings, and improved wage standards for employees. How were they to pay for this, when everybody seemed to be demanding to get backlogged services at the old prices?

For centuries, hospitals had existed on a system of collecting whatever they could, and delivering needed care as best they were able. Their deficits were covered by public subscription, by religions, and by tightening the belts of the charity minded hospital volunteers. Sometimes the rich guy who lived in a mansion on the hill would donate, sometimes he wouldn't. Surely, the government had a responsibility to rescue such a deserving charity. The student nurses and the young doctors in white, worked for no pay at all. That's right, after I graduated from medical school I worked for four years without a dime of pay. If hospitals overcharged a few insurance companies, well, there was nothing else they could do to keep the doors open. Until health insurance made a significant impact, hospitals ruled medical care. They were the only institutions which seemed to work, all new ideas seemed to come from them, and any new idea which came along was somehow centered within hospitals. Although it wasn't described as such, hospitals began to suffer the disease of conglomerates. If an organization takes on too many functions at once, it performs some of them poorly. Usually, one of the subsidiaries fails and drags the rest of the conglomerate down. That's essentially why the Supreme Court, in the *State Oil v. Khan* case finally decided vertical integration cures itself and usually does not require antitrust judicial action to break it up. That doesn't mean vertical integration is wonderful; it just has to be shown to be bad before you punish it. Unfortunately, high legal fees unbalance the situation. The corporation can usually afford the lawyers, the individual practitioner can't. Threatening to bankrupt the opponent is now a standard procedure in the courts of Justice.

Disregard for the Tenth Amendment in the 1937 Court-packing incident greatly injured the Tenth Amendment's Constitutional requirement that health and health-related activities should be regulated at the state level. But it also heightened public attention on the Constitutional issue, since hospitals, nurses, doctors, pharmacies, and the Blue Cross organizations were all organized along state lines. Only when the Federal government under Harry Truman began to sound serious about central control of medical care, did health insurance begin to cross state lines, and thus weakened hospital and Blue Cross domination of it. By the time Lyndon Johnson began his piecemeal assault in 1965 with Medicare and Medicaid, the insurance industry had broken healthcare into four "markets":

Large-employer groups. The healthiest groups, and hence the cheapest to insure, became the low-hanging fruit. Union pressure combined with the passage of ERISA, expanded and somewhat fragmented the groups, but large employers were first and dominant in the planning.

Small-employer groups. Curiously, this often became the most expensive silo of the markets, because of successful pressure to expand – even mandate – benefit packages, and the fact that certain expensive cost generators can be selectively insured when the personnel manager knows them by name.

Individuals. Because of adverse self-selection, "non-group" had the highest marketing costs, and often the highest medical costs. It was possible to eliminate the worst abuses, such as figuratively buying insurance while riding to the hospital in an ambulance. But subscribers to non-group insurance move freely between employers, and thus can avoid being dropped from the insurance when they change jobs. What is generally touted as a great disadvantage of employer-based insurance, could easily be called an exploitation of being in a position to select only healthy people for jobs. Insurance companies obviously and regularly "prefer to work with groups". Circumvention wears many disguises. When an insurer tells you this is "his company's policy", be sure to kick him in the shins. His company is part of the problem, not part of the solution.

Executive "Cadillac" plans. are mentioned for completeness, although they could also be grouped with steak dinners and baseball tickets, as mere sales promotion kickbacks for the people who make decisions on behalf of members of a large group. They often had "first dollar coverage", essentially paying for everything even faintly describable as medical care, down to the last penny. It should prompt some concern to learn that health insurance for college professors and politicians is often of this variety. In terms of aggregate medical cost, or course, Cadillac plans are negligible. However, as long as they exist, they light the way for those fortunates who can focus on Henry Kaiser gimmicks rather than the treatment of illness, and eventually migrate to the rest of the tax-deductible group.

The general purpose of market stratification is to offer much the same product at different prices. Like other concessions which vice makes to virtue, they constrain admiration for the essential, desirable, feature of insurance in the first place: it spreads the risk and lessens the cost of what is supposedly an unpredictable random health catastrophe. If the insurance industry is really serious about this mission, it would start with one outstanding example of it: catastrophic coverage. Remember, the higher the deductible, the lower the premium. Let's repeat that: the higher the deductible, the lower the premium. Are insurance companies really motivated to have lower premiums? That's like saying Insurance Companies want to lower legal costs in order to preserve the impartiality of the courts.

Almost nobody can withstand a million-dollar illness, but almost anybody can afford a hundred dollars a year. Once you have that minimum feature, you can then start to talk about more expensive, more common coverage – until we eventually reach first-dollar coverage for non-essentials, at wildly unaffordable premiums. By the way, if you would like to know why I didn't acquire catastrophic coverage back in the days when it was widely available, it was because I already had first-dollar coverage given to me by the University where I worked, I couldn't use extra catastrophic coverage even if it was free. This is no longer pre-1965. Everyone should have catastrophic coverage. Only if he can afford it, should anyone have more than that. Since the logic is beyond dispute, has it occurred to anyone to ask why that isn't the usual case? Read on.

Henry Kaiser's Cleverness Out of Control

The Henry Kaiser caper. In 1943 during the Second World War, Henry Kaiser was given "Liberty Ship" contracts to build freighters for the Pacific Theater. To build ships in East Coast shipyards was to invite German U-boats to sink them as they headed for the Panama Canal. There was a price-control mandate from the War Production Board, seeking to restrain wartime inflation by prohibiting raises or bonuses. So Kaiser protested he had difficulty attracting steelworkers to California because he could not offer incentives to move. By whatever means of persuasion, Kaiser was able to obtain an exemption, permitting him to treat healthcare fringe benefits as non-salary, thus exempt from income taxation. As Cicero noticed, "In times of war, the Law falls silent." Other expedients may have been allowed, just in order to win the war, but such loopholes were apparently closed after victory was achieved. This one persisted.

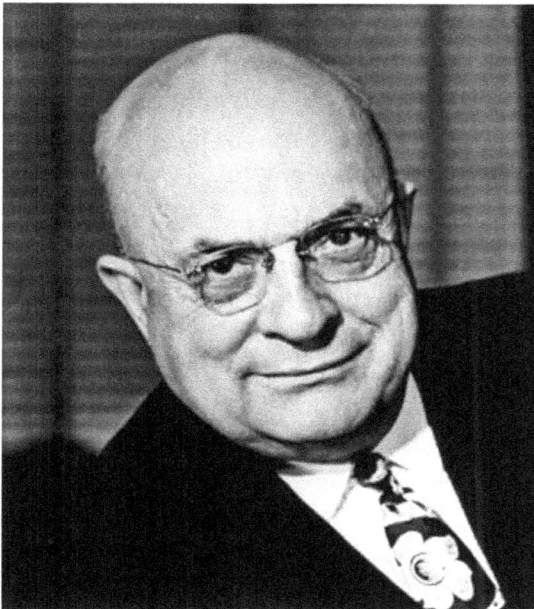

Henry J. Kaiser

In later post-war years, just exactly who negotiated with whom remains unclear, but in essence the IRS continued to treat employer health benefits as tax-exempt gifts, and still does, eighty years later – provided the employer pays the premium. This unintended post-war extension is fiercely defended by organized labor whenever someone brings it up, and they are quietly supported by the managements of big business. Congressmen are scared of the whole subject because of bad experiences with united lobbying, linking unions and big business. In Washington, such an alliance unites the support of the leaders of both political parties. It must be mentioned here that Government itself is one of the biggest beneficiaries, acting as a huge

> *"The ones carrying the placards, are seldom running the show."*
> **Protest Politics**

employer offering fringe benefits, itself. Consequently, Congress itself finds it has a conflict of interest when the subject is on the floor.

The central feature is, the employer must give a gift of insurance to the employee; self-employed and unemployed persons are not entitled to it, nor would employees be, if they bought it for themselves. After a while economists agree the gift becomes an accepted part of the wage cost and the pay packet gradually falls to adjust for it. However, other taxes and charges are based as a percent of wages, and so the gift results in even greater tax benefit than the same amount in wages would. How long it takes for wages to adjust an equivalent amount can be argued, but after eighty years, it is safe to say they are fully adjusted. Since the corporate income tax is about double the individual rate, the savings to the employer are appreciably greater than the savings to the employee.

Clamor to retain this tax ruse is joined by non-profit charities and state, local and federal businesses, who are included in the favored tax-excluded group – even though it would appear the employers do not share in this feature. Their revenues are often fixed, and their budgets have shifted to expect this gift; consequently their noise is equally loud when discontinuation is suggested. My own medical society employees participate. As James Madison feared when he designed the Constitution, the number in the wagon being pulled outnumber the people pulling the wagon. In the lobbying case, the ones carrying the placards are seldom the ones running the show, and seldom fully understand the issue.

Small businesses are entitled to the tax exemption but many do not avail themselves of the opportunity when they discover premium rates for their group of employees are often higher than the individual rate. Furthermore, small businesses are overall less dependably profitable than big ones, so their tax rates are usually lower. The essence of the self-interest of big business for "employee" health benefits tends to concentrate in those companies who make big profits, and thus pay high corporate taxes; less profitable businesses have less tax liability to play games with. Things take time to emerge, but after eighty years there has been plenty of time for the "gift" to be taken for granted, and the pay packet gradually adjusted to recognize that fact. Nothing remains to justify it except the tax deduction.

While it is hard to be precise, it is obvious that when things get less expensive they attract more buyers. Generally speaking, higher-wage businesses have lower health insurance premiums, because they can be more selective in their hiring, partly as a consequence of lower costs in their experience rating. Moreover, if an employee somehow gets a gift of

> *"Gifts to employees are more tax-sheltered than equivalent salary would be."*

his insurance premium, his employer actually saves more than he does, although less attention gets drawn to it. If there is anything a big business gets fierce about, it is to be deprived of savings which seem to result from its own cleverness. In this case, that argument seems more acceptable than it really is, since the benefit is now almost exclusively sustained by lobbying. The employee would have had to pay a higher income tax on a higher salary if he bought his own insurance with after-tax dollars. But that tax is based on his gross before-tax cost, including Social Security, Medicare, and other assessments, which the employer pays less of, on a lowered salary. Nor must he pay half of this and half of that, itemized on the pay stub, in matching money. This part of his cost is reduced by about 35% when he gives away the health insurance, and everything else is a tax wash. That is, other taxes have been warped to take advantage of the tax exclusion, with the result the employer community is not entirely unwilling to have unions demand they be coordinated that way.

The overall result is both employee and employer are better off than by just a straight tax deduction on the insurance premium, while the employer is far better off because he can multiply it by the number of his employees. Google, for example, has 55,000 employees, some of whom are paid extraordinary salaries. And then, the employer's tax deduction is against a 40% tax rate instead of against a blended tax rate for the employees of perhaps 20%. And finally, the insurance premium is reduced below the individual rate by forming a group and demanding hospital discounts. All of this is the result of gifting health insurance premiums on behalf of the employees. For executives with an very high salary, it can probably accomplish remarkable savings for the shareholders by giving the executive a Cadillac plan. Because it makes a good smoke-screen, no one troubles to correct wide-spread misapprehensions, especially among others who are already tax-exempt.

Indeed, a little multiplication is convincing that tax abatement is not only supporting a substantial proportion of health insurance, but it represents a noticeable portion of corporate profits. So, although a major portion of this distortion would soon readjust to a new climate of opinion, any move in the direction of removing it abruptly would probably unnerve the stock market for an indeterminate time. It took eighty years to build up to this condition, and it cannot be corrected in a few days. It would therefore be important to have a solution to it, ready to be announced. Here's my proposal.

> **Proposal 4:** That a schedule of reduction of both the tax exemption of employer-based health insurance <u>and</u> the corporate income tax be prepared along the following lines: That in consultation with economists, the corporate income tax rate be reduced until it matches the average blended individual tax rate. <u>And</u> the tax exemption for employer-based health insurance be reduced in a step-wise fashion, until it disappears. The process shall take no longer than three (3) tax years, keep the two reductions in balance, and be commented upon by the Federal Reserve, and overseen by an appropriate committee of both House and Senate.

While it is conventional to ascribe a tax evasion to the employee, and to blame it on those dreadful unions, the employer gets somewhat more tax benefit than each employee, multiplied by thousands of employees in the bigger firms – but it's just a tax dodge for both shareholders and employees, with the shareholders coming out somewhat ahead. Nevertheless, the employer advantage mostly derives from comparing an individual employee gain with an aggregated corporation gain. It may reflect union salesmanship that the aggregate employee gain is usually not displayed, since that immediately makes the two more nearly equal.

Since salesmanship has come up, I might as well apply a little of it to my own proposal. I believe sober analysis reaches the conclusion that the tax exemption is about all that matters, to anyone. Following the proposal, the government would gain taxes and corporation stakeholders would have to pay them. The shareholders would be compensated by a corporate tax reduction, but the employees would not. Although the employer might argue either side, the employees would be the ones who would surely complain. But let's take it another step.

Let's recall what happened in Ireland when the corporate tax rate was reduced to 12.5% in 1983 from its former rate of 50% in 1982. Essentially nothing happened to government revenue, which has only varied at much as 10% between 1975 and 2015. There was hardly a ripple in 1983. That's not to say nothing happened, it just did not affect government revenue much. For that to be the case, it is mathematically necessary to have more corporations, each paying less tax. That's indeed what seemed to happen, but it took twenty years to convulse the Irish economy, starting from a comparatively low level. Ireland is mostly a rural nation, and new corporations came in from abroad (UK and Scandinavia, mostly) to locate primarily in Dublin, as city dwellers. That started a housing boom, which required mortgages, and eventually toppled the banks. The Irish corporate tax rates remained at 12.5% before, during and after the crash. The present American state and federal tax rate is the highest in the world, and our situation is that corporations are fleeing abroad to escape it. The corporate tax refugees in Ireland have so far generally remained in Ireland, probably because it is disruptive to move and the people speak English.

Judging by the Irish experience, America could similarly expect the fundamentals might change more slowly than might be guessed, but probably more quickly than they did in Ireland. The net effect on government revenues would be negligible, but the effect on employment would be strikingly positive. With higher employment, wages would rise. Somebody would lose, but it wouldn't be America; a deft new President might even be able to deploy some new power abroad, peacefully but firmly.

The current President might have to ride a bucking broncho for a few weeks. So in summary, most of the economic turmoil to be feared would likely be short-term and in the financial markets. I can easily imagine the scepticism with which the affected employees would greet this analysis, and all the op-ed columns in the usual newspapers. Balanced against that, American medical care would at least get a lot of distortion wrung out of its accounting processes, and surely would be improved in the long run, by regaining control of its own finances.

Let's return to the details. It is sometimes argued the gift of insurance premiums is an addition to the salary, but almost all economists agree the salary soon re-adjusts up or down, to reappear in the pay packet. Stop calling it wages and treat it as <u>total wage costs</u>, and you soon see the point. No doubt it takes time to adjust, and it seems fair to say the employer benefits from corporate tax reduction more quickly than the individual employee does. The tax amount comes close to $2000 per year per employee. Because the hidden benefit lies in taxes, the profitability of the company enters in as well, and what is true of one employer may not be as true of another. In particular, it is not true of the government and non-profit sectors, who have no corporate income taxes to pay. There may be some political hope in that.

If a business is profitable to the full limit of corporate taxes, the nominal benefit is the full limit of the employee's tax bracket, but the offset to the employer can be about twice that rate in corporate taxes. Here, we assume a blended income tax rate of 20% for the employee, and 39% top state and federal rates for the employer. In companies with 10,000 employees the financial saving alone can be considerable. Almost all corporations listed on an exchange are profitable most of the time; there might be more swing in smaller businesses.

Anyway, sometimes it just seems more attractive for small businesses to have Subchapter S tax treatment. On that subject, it is a little difficult to say what pressures motivate small family businesses. Some people allege the whole Subchapter S complexity is a reaction to utilizing this distinction, and therefore should be counted as an indirect benefit of the Henry Kaiser gambit. During the 2009 Tea Party agitations however, it was noticeable that small businessmen at the microphone were extremely vocal in their opposition to Obamacare. Unfortunately, it is hard to know how well small business understands the inside operations of big businesses. As they say, Macy's doesn't tell Gimbels.

With regard to all employees as a class, it seems safe to say people who are well enough to be employed, have mostly lower healthcare costs, and therefore seem more attractive in the eyes of their health insurance company. That would maybe result in lower premiums. Since only 25% of persons aged 25-34 are insured, Obamacare calculated they would break even if they enrolled 40% of the "young invincibles" at average rates. Generally speaking, that would be males, who – without the Henry Kaiser gimmick – might have an 80% avoidance rate. But remember, there's also the automobile insurance phenomenon: compulsory auto insurance induces a great many to stop paying premiums after the first month or two.

With Obamacare, the dropout rate is reported to be 13% during the first year of operation. The kids resent being overcharged for something they feel they don't need, and calling them "young invincibles" inflames rather than softens that feeling. The much more important point is **they don't get anything back when they are older**, except sympathy. That's the central flaw in employer-based one-year term insurance, and let's hope you notice the Health Savings Account corrects the injustice. With auto accidents, young people have higher rates, and that's accepted as normal. With health insurance following the same logic, it ought to be the other way around, shouldn't it?

Taken all together, it is pretty easy to see why big business demanded a one-year exempted delay from Obamacare, which later was extended another year. No doubt they intend to keep a low profile, but will keep demanding "temporary" exemptions, at least until the recession is over, and possibly forever. Until we see the eventual experience with employees, the largest group affected, it will be impossible to predict the limits of the subsidy program for the uninsured. Nevertheless, it is fairly obvious this essentially political impasse is being treated as an untouchable issue, and believable estimations of "fairness" will be a long time in coming. Businesses of all sizes like to present themselves as a big happy family. But in fact the large common market produced by our continental boundaries means a comparatively small amount of American trade (but admittedly a growing one) is international. The main competition for big American business is small American business, and don't you forget it.

To a fairly large extent, this split is also a split between family-controlled business and stockholder-controlled business, between Subchapter S and Subchapter C corporations, and between university-educated management and small-college educated bosses. It's geographic, it's regional; it's R and it's D. If you ever watched a pro football game with businessmen in the audience, you know both large ones and small ones always feel challenged, and both intend to win, even when they might both end up losing.

Solutions: Nevertheless, the issue of revenue neutrality, at least for employer-based health insurance, is easily summarized. You don't have to be a professional negotiator to see that something close to a 2/3 exemption for everybody could make it revenue neutral. And then, through inflation and other traditional means of attrition, mid-course corrections might whittle it down.

But that's only part of it. Remember, the employee payroll deduction is only half of the issue. The employer gets the other half, by paying lower corporate taxes. His total payroll cost ends up much the same, but by this time the reader should see that doesn't matter. Corporate taxes are too high, probably in part because of class antagonisms. We have a flight of corporations abroad, and we see the Irish example that you shouldn't go too fast. But a reassuring part of this problem is we have Congress to negotiate it. Having learned how to raise food stamps by raising farm subsidies, they don't need any lessons in triangulation. No need to mention volume discounts on the insurance premiums, and discounts the insurance company shifts to the hospital. The details of such features are not public information.

Taken altogether, it sometimes appears equal treatment might be easier to attain than elimination of the tax exemption. If everyone received a tax exemption, at least in part, we might at least eliminate the distortions imposed by rent-seeking the loopholes. It might raise healthcare prices at a time we need to lower them, so a stepwise approach might turn out to be the only feasible one. This is a time when healthcare is so expensive that only a really radical approach might be noticeable. Perhaps it is time just to get rid of the inequality, so later sacrifices for economy will not seem so hypocritical.

There's one other misconception to be wary of. A tax reduction at the 50% employer rate is not at all the same as a 50% reduction of the employer's taxes, although it may sound like it. It's likely to be far smaller.

Public Misconceptions

(Healthcare for Citizen Lobbyists)

There are a few other ideas about the cost of medical care, which I would say are widely held, but the truth of which seems dubious. In fact, I would characterize them as misconceptions. If misconceptions are held long enough, they eventually work their way into the tax code.

Is Preventive Medicine Always and Everywhere Less Expensive? As heads nod vigorously in support of prevention, please notice in general usage it suggests several different things. The overall implication is that small interventions for everyone are less expensive to society; less expensive, that is, than large expenses for the few who get the disease. That is clearly not invariably the case, and unfortunately in a compulsory insurance world, it may seldom be the case. The point is not that preventive care is a bad thing, because it is often a very good thing, even by far the very best thing. It's just not necessarily cheaper.

Take for example a tetanus toxoid booster, which ten years ago cost less than a dollar for the material. Recently in preparation for a vacation trip, I was charged $85 dollars by my corner drugstore, just for the material. If you do the math, $85.00 times millions of Americans is a far greater sum than the present aggregate cost of Americans actually contracting tetanus, especially following the advice to have a booster shot every ten years. This becomes more certain if one adds in the cost of administration. The vaccine is quite effective, Americans had almost

> *"Better, yes.*
> *Cheaper? No."*
> **Preventive**
> **Medicine**

no cases in the Far Eastern Theater in World War II. The British who did not vaccinate routinely, had large numbers of often fatal cases. Furthermore, even if the tetanus patient survives, the disease is hideously painful. Is it better to immunize routinely? **Yes, it is.** Is it cheaper? I'm not entirely sure, because I have no access to production costs of tetanus toxoid. But it certainly seems likely it isn't cheaper. Malpractice costs, which are a different issue entirely, complicate this opinion.

Something, probably malpractice liability, has transformed an effective preventive procedure from clearly cost effective to – probably not cheaper for a nation which no longer has horses on the streets, but still has horses on farms and ranches. This is presently mostly a malpractice liability problem for the vaccine maker, not a preventive care issue. Take another well-known example. In the case of smallpox vaccination, it is now clearly more expensive to vaccinate everyone in the world than to treat the few actual cases. The waffle currently being employed is to limit vaccination to countries where there are still a few cases, hoping thereby to eradicate the disease from the planet.

Over and over, examination of individual vaccinations shows the answer to be: better, yes, cheaper, no; with the ultimate answer depending on accounting tricks in the calculation of cost, cost inflation because of third-party payment, and related perplexities. To be measured about it, excessive profitability of some preventive measures could act as a stimulant for finally calling off prevention, by taking on a briefly more expensive campaign to achieve final eradication. Somewhere in this issue is the whisper that "natural" gene diversity of any sort must never be totally eliminated, a viewpoint which even the diversity philosopher William James never openly extended to include virulent diseases

Routine cervical pap tests, routine annual physical examinations, routine colonoscopies and a host of other routines are in general open to questioning as to cost effectiveness. The issue is likely to increase rather than go away. Much of the current denunciation of "Cadillac" health insurance plans focuses on the elaborate prevention programs enjoyed by Wall Street executives, college professors, industrial unions, and other privileged health insurance classes. A more useful approach to a borderline issue might focus on removing such items from health insurance benefit packages, particularly those whose cost is subsidized, either directly or by income tax deductions. Those preventive measures which demonstrate cost effectiveness can have their subsidy restored, or be grouped together into a category which must compete for eligible access to limited funds.

The inference is strong that unrestrained substitution of community prevention for patient treatment escalates costs rather considerably, and – at the least – needs to demonstrate more cost effectiveness before subsidy is extended. While self-interest is a possibility if only physicians are consulted, total reliance on bean-counters could eliminate benevolent judgment entirely. Community cost effectiveness is a ratio, and both sides must be fairly argued. Don't forget many people quietly recognize the need for gigantic cost-shifting between age groups. Spending money on young workers to pay for shots is one way to shift the cost of elderly illness, backwards to the employer they no longer work for. It can be a pretty expensive way to do it.

In the final analysis, without some form of patient participation in the cost, this issue is probably unsolvable. To launch a host of double-blind clinical trials to find out the truth will lead to answers of some sort, which will quickly be undermined by price/cost confusion, leading to increasingly futile regulation. Including preventive costs in the deductible at least allows public participation in the decisions and true balance to begin; which is to say, even universal preventive care admiration cannot be adequately assessed except in the presence of a substantial open market for the product.

Much "preventive" care is really "early detection" or "early management". That's entirely different. When the goal changes so subtly, it is often not possible to judge what is worthwhile, except by placing some price on pain and suffering. The abuse by the trial bar of the monetization of pain and suffering in the malpractice field, ought to be a gentle reminder of that. Preventive colonoscopy has clearly caused a decline in deaths from colon cancer; that's a medical judgment, and a transitional one. Whether the cost of catching those cancers early was cost effective is largely a matter of colonoscopy cost, and on digging into it, will be found to be as much an anesthesia issue as a colonoscopist one. In any event, it is not one where the opinion of insurance

> *"Average Hospital Profit Margins: Inpatient 2%, Accident Room 15%, Satellite Clinics 30%"*
> **Payment by Diagnosis**

reviewers should be decisive. If the litigation industry moves to make omission of prevention a new source of action, it will surely be a sign it is past time, to caution the public about the direction of things.

Outpatient is Not Necessarily Cheaper Than Inpatient For the Same Problem. Medicare provides half of hospital revenue; the other half is often dragged into a uniform approach. The reimbursement mostly has nothing to do with the itemized bills hospitals send, and may have little to do with production costs. The DRG (Diagnosis-Related Groups) system for reimbursing hospitals *for inpatients* is thus not directly based on specific costs in the inpatient area. It is related to clustered diagnoses lumped into a DRG group, and then assumes overpayments will eventually balance underpayments within individual hospitals.

That last point, depending on the Law of Large Numbers, is questionable, and especially so in small hospitals. When two million diagnoses are condensed into 200 Diagnosis groups, group uniformity just has to be uneven. Reimbursement means repayment, but this interposed step often interferes with that definition. Someone in the past fifty years discovered the reimbursement step was an excellent choke point. Manipulating the reimbursement rates without changing the service is a handy place to choose winners and losers; it's largely out of sight of the people who would recognize it for what it is.

Furthermore, for various DRG groups, or for all of them, it becomes possible to construct a fairly tight rationing system for inpatient costs.

The degree to which actual production costs match a particular DRG reimbursement rate, is blurred by inevitable imprecision in the DRG code construction. It is impossible to squash a couple of million diagnoses into two hundred code numbers without imprecision. It works both ways, of course. The coders back at the hospital will seek weaknesses out, experimentally. A grossly generalized code is placed in the hands of hospital employees, resulting in a system which suits both sides of the transaction, but is one which ought to be abolished, on both sides, by computerizing the process. At least, computers could avoid the issue of mistranslating the doctors' English into code.

The overall outcome with Medicare is an average 2% profit margin on inpatients during a 2% national inflation. This is far too tight to expect it to come out precisely right for everybody. And in fact, inflation has averaged 3% for a century, but is 1.6% right now. The Federal Reserve Chairman desperately tries to raise it, but it just won't go up. If you don't think this is a serious issue, just reflect that our gold-less currency is supported by a 2% inflation target which the Federal Reserve is proving unable to maintain.

For technical reasons, the same forced loss is not true of outpatient and emergency services, which usually use Chargemaster values. Emergency services are said to approximate 15% profit margins, and outpatient services, 30%. It is therefore difficult to believe anyone would start anywhere but the profit margin, and work backward to managing the institution. In consequence the buyer's intermediary has stolen the pricing process from the seller. Without the need to communicate one word, prices rise to the level of available payment, and then stop there. But let's not be too specific in our suspicions. Some incentive to direct patients to the emergency and outpatient areas must develop, and is acted upon in the pricing. It just doesn't have to be so confusing and so high-handed.

Any assumption by the public that outpatient care is cheaper than inpatient hospital care is likely to be quite misleading. Short of driving the hospital out of business, revenue in this system is whatever the insurance intermediary chooses to make it. There was a time when the intermediary was Blue Cross, and behind them, big business. Nowadays, it is Medicare, but Obamacare probably aspires to the turf.

Let's test the reasoning by using different data. Because hospital inpatient care is reimbursed at roughly 106% of overall cost, while hospital outpatient care is reimbursed at roughly 150%, hospitals are impelled to favor outpatient care, no matter which type of care happens to have the cheapest production cost, the best medical outcomes, or enjoys the greatest comforts. Instead, the rates and ratios are ultimately determined by magazine articles and newspaper editorials. At some level within the government, a political system responds to what it thinks is public opinion, *vox populi est vox dei.* No matter what their personal feelings may be, hospital management encounters more quarrelsomeness on wages in the inpatient area, less resistance in the outpatient and home care programs. So, true costs must actually rise in the outpatient area, sooner or later, following the financial incentives. Personnel shortages follow, as does friction between hospitals and office-based physicians. The process is circular, but the origin of favoring outpatient care over inpatient care was primarily driven by some accountant reading a magazine article.

A highly similar attitude underlies the hubub for salaried physicians rather than fee-for service. It's a short-cut to a forty-hour week, and following that, to a doctor shortage. And following that, to enlarged medical school budgets. If anyone imagines that will save money, the reasoning is obscure.

Everybody can guess what it costs to wash a couple of sheets and buy a couple of TV dinners. Everyone fundamentally understands Society's need to transfer medical costs from the sick population to the well population. Nothing known about hotel prices justifies a 50% difference in price between inpatient and outpatient care, all else being equal. The room price mainly supports overhead costs which are unrelated to direct patient care, so those fixed costs are like migratory birds, settling to roost where it's quiet. Remember, it isn't costs driving the system, it is now profit margins.

The Return of a Discharged Hospital Patient Within 30 Days is not Necessarily a Sign of Bad Care. Rather, it reflects the fact that hospital inpatient reimbursement is entirely based on the bulk number of admissions, not the sum of itemized ingredients. Having undermined fee for service, Medicare must resort to taxing the whole admission.

Early re-admission can of course be a sign of premature discharge or careless coordination with the home physician. But these issues are so remote from the basic reason for admission, that bulk punishment is unlikely to change the criticized behavior. That behavior may mean a convalescent center is convenient to a hospital, making it reasonable to move the patient without much loss of continuity of care; and treating his return to the acute facility becomes a matter of small consequence. It is also a matter of cost accounting; when you claim a hundred dollar hotel cost to be worth thousands of dollars, many distortions are inevitable. If a hospital essentially shuts down on weekends, for example, there actually might be better care available somewhere else.

Imposing a penalty for returns to the hospital post-discharge, has certainly changed behavior, but it is far from clear whether institutions are better as a result. Without a detailed study of longitudinal effects and costs, this threat is no more than an untested experiment. Without access to accounting practices, doctors assume the penalty for a high re-admission rate merely affirms that hospital insurance reimbursement by DRG is solely dependent on the discharge diagnosis, therefore bears little relation to the quality of care. Given a particular diagnosis, reimbursement is totally independent of any other cost. When all you have is a hammer, everything looks like a nail to the DRG.

The legitimate reasons for re-admission to the hospital are many and varied. Collectively, they could well constitute a general attitude on the part of a particular hospital that it is reasonable to send many patients home a little early in order to achieve greater overall cost savings – in spite of sustaining a few re-admissions. But this is somewhat beside the point. The insurance companies accept the fallacy that favoring readmission is the only way a hospital can increase reimbursement under a DRG system. This is merely a debater's trick of redefining the issue, from true cost to reimbursement amount. More or fewer tests, longer or shorter stays have no effect, but readmission cans double reimbursement. Consequently, re-admission has been stigmatized as invariably signifying careless treatment, justifying a penalty reduction of overall reimbursement. This is high-handed, indeed. It would require a research project to determine which of the alleged motives is actually operational.

The Doughnut Hole: Deductibles versus Copayments. To understand why the doughnut hole is a good idea, you have to understand why copay is a flawed idea. In both cases, the purpose is to make the patient responsible for some of the cost in order to restrain abuse. As the expression goes, you want the patient to have some skin in the game. The question is how to do it; the doughnut has not been widely tried, but the copayment approach is very familiar: charge the patient 20% of the cost, in cash.

This co-pay idea finds great favor with management and labor in negotiations, because the premium savings are immediately known. If the copayment is 10%, then employer cost will be decreased 10%; if it is 50%, the cost is reduced 50%. In midnight bargaining sessions, such simplicity is much appreciated. However, the doughnut hole was not devised to make negotiations simpler for group insurance, it was devised to inhibit reckless spending, theoretically unleashed once the initial deductible has been satisfied.

Health insurance companies also like both co-pay and doughnuts for questionable reasons. Both offer an opportunity to sell two insurance policies as two pieces of the same patient encounter, adding up to 100% coverage, but eliminating the patient's skin in the game. Doubling the marketing and administrative fees seems like an advantage only to an insurance intermediary, while it totally undermines the incentive of restraining patient overuse. In practice, having two insurances for every charge has led to mysterious delays in payment of the second one, even though they are often administered by the same company. Physicians and other providers hate the system, not only because it involves two insurance claims processes per claim, but because it often makes it impossible to calculate the residual after insurance, i.e., patient cash responsibility, until months after the service has been rendered. Patients often take this long silence to imply payment in full, and disputes with the provider are common. Long ago, older physicians warned the younger ones, "Always collect your fees while the tears are hot."

It has long been a mystery why hospital bills take so long to go through the system; at one time, protracting the interest float seemed a plausible motive. However, the persistence of delayed processing during a period of near-zero interest rates makes this motive unlikely. It now occurs to me that the reimbursement of health insurance costs by the business employer is related to corporate tax payments, and hence to the quarterly tax system. Using the puzzling model of a monthly bank statement for online reporting would have some logic, but great confusion, attached to the bank statement approach for group payment utility. But in the end, I really do not understand why health insurance reimbursement or even reporting to the patient, should take so many months, and cause so much difficulty. Recently, the major insurance companies have started to imitate banks by putting the monthly statement continuously online on the Internet. If doctors find a way to be notified, the billing cycle could be speeded up considerably, and even the deplorable custom of demanding cash in advance may abate. The intermediaries probably won't do it, so it is a business opportunity for some software company, and a minor convenience for the group billing clerk.

So, the idea of a doughnut hole was born, after empirical observation about what was owed on two levels, one for small common claims, and another for big ones. Formerly, the patient either paid cash in full or was insured in full, so arriving at the Paradise of full coverage is purchased in cash within the first deductible. Unfortunately, once that last threshold was crossed, the sky became the limit. Some way really had to be found to distinguish between extravagant over-use, and the use of highly expensive drugs, particularly those still under patent protection. The idea was generated that if the two levels of the doughnut hole were calculated from actual claims data, there might often be a clear separation of minor illnesses from major ones. Since the patient would ordinarily be uncertain how far he was from triggering the doughnut hole, the restraint of abuse might carry over, even into areas where the facts were not as feared.

It is too early to judge the relative effectiveness of the two different patient-responsibility approaches, but it is not too early to watch politicians pander to confusion caused by an innovative but unfamiliar approach, while the insurance administrators simplify their own task by applying a general rule, instead of tailoring it to the service or drug. And by the way, the patients who complain so bitterly about a novel insurance innovation, are deprived by the donut hole of a way to maintain "first-dollar" coverage, which is a major cause of the cost inflations they also complain so much about. Some people think they can fix any problem just by loudly complaining about it. Perhaps, in a politicized situation, it works; but it doesn't fool anyone.

Plan Design. The insurance industry, particularly the actuaries working in that area, have long and sophisticated experience with the considerations leading to upper and lower limits, exclusions and exceptions. Legislative committees would be wise to solicit advice on these matters, which ordinarily have little political content. However, the advisers from the insurance world have an eye to bidding on later contracts to advise and administer these plans. They are not immune to the temptation to advise inclusion of provisions which invisibly slant the contract toward a particular bidder, and failing that, they look for ways to make things easier, or more profitable, for whichever insurance company does get the contract. The doughnut hole is a recent example of these incentives in action; no member of any congressional committee was able to explain the doughnut for a television audience, so it was ridiculed. The outcome has been a race between politicians to see who could most quickly figure out a way to reduce the size of the hole. The idea that the size of the hole was intended to be an automatic adjustment to experience, seems to have been totally lost in the shuffle. Asking industry experts for advice is fine, but it would be well to ask for such advice from several other sources, too.

Fee-for-Service Billing. In recent years, a number of my colleagues have taken up the idea that fee-for-service billing is a bad thing, possibly the root of all evil. Just about everyone who says this, is himself working for a salary; and I suspect it is a pre-fabricated argument to justify that method of payment. The obvious retort is that if you do more work, you ought to be paid more. The pre-fabricated Q and A goes on to reply, this is how doctors "game" the system, by embroidering a little. I suppose that is occasionally the case, but the conversation seems so stereotyped, I take it to be a soft-spoken way of accusing me of being a crook, so I usually explode with some ill-considered counter-attack. My basic position is that the patient has considerable responsibility to act protectively on his own behalf. That is unfortunately often undermined by excessive or poorly-designed health insurance. Nobody washes a rental car, because that's considered to be the responsibility of the car rental agency. A more serious flaw in the argument that we should eliminate fee for service, was taught me in Canada.

When Canada adopted socialized medicine, I was asked to go there by my medical society, to see what it was all about. That put me in conversation with a number of Canadian hospital administrators, and the conversation skipped around among common topics. Since I was interested in cost-accounting as the source of much of our problems, I asked how they managed. Well, as soon as paying for hospital care became a provincial responsibility, they stopped preparing itemized bills. Consequently, it immediately became impossible to tell how much anything cost. The administrator knew what he bought, and he paid the bills for the hospital. But how much was spent on gall bladder surgery or obstetrics, he wouldn't be in a position to know.

So I took up the same subject with the Canadian doctors, who reported the same problem in a different form. Given a choice of a surgical treatment or a medical one for the same condition, they simply did not know which one was cheaper. After a while, the hospital charges were abandoned as a method of telling what costs more, and eventually no effort was made to determine comparative prices at all. There's no sense in an American getting smug about this, because manipulation of the DRG soon divorced hospital billing charges from having any relation to underlying costs, and American doctors soon gave up any effort to use billing as a guide to treatment choices. We organize task forces to generate "typical" bills from time to time, but these standardized cost analyses are a crude and expensive substitute for the immediacy of a particular patient's bill.

My friends in the Legal Profession make a sort of similar complaint. The advent of cheap computers created the concept of "billable hours", in which some fictional average price is fixed to a two-minute phone consultation. In the old days, my friends tell me, they always would have a conference with the client, just before sending a bill. The client was asked how much he thought the services were worth to him, and often the figure was higher than the actual bill. In the cases where the conjectured price was lower, the attorney had an opportunity to explain the cleverness of his maneuvers, or the time-consuming effort required to develop the evidence. A senior attorney told me that never in his life did he send a bill for more than the client agreed to pay, and he was a happier man for it. Naturally, the bills were higher when the attorney won the case than when he lost it, which is definitely not the case when a hospital is unsuccessful in a cancer cure. Similarly, you might think bills would be higher if the patient lived than if he died, but income maximization always takes the higher choice. So the absence of this face-to-face discussion is a regrettable one in medical care, as well.

Hospital Cost-Shifting by Age Group, Patient Income, and Payer Class

When kids get sick, the parents pay the costs. When the grandparents get sick, Medicare may well pay a large part out of tax withholdings, premiums and government borrowing, but working children still are the last resort for the grandparent generation, if resources fail. What's the common theme, here?

All medical costs, whatever the age of the patient, ultimately rest on the contributions of some working person, aged 21 to 66. The medical payment system is largely driven toward transferring funds from non-sick people to sickly non-working ones. The non-sick increasingly resent this stubborn fact, but as long as we continue an employer-based system it will only get worse. It is necessarily a dangerous hostility to encourage.

Indeed, our whole society is somewhat based on the interdependent family unit, using the assumption breadwinners pay for themselves and children, and are ultimately responsible for their parents as well. It's somewhat dismaying to reflect, that with a decline in the power of religion, a decline of importance of the family may threaten the stability of many under-examined issues, just like healthcare financing. If the employer or the government supersede the family, the family is still the fall-back; and anyway, all taxes and profits ultimately derive from working people, just not the family's own, particular, working people.

Whole generations vocalize decreased respect for marriage in various ways, but do not seem to have considered the disruption it would cause, to get taken at their word. Viewed both ways, if we discuss the ability to pay for healthcare, we have to admit there is nobody to stand behind those bills, whatever the age of the patient – except some breadwinner. Then, when we ask whether the country can support the cost of healthcare, we are actually questioning whether a solitary age generation of workers can really afford to pay the current costs of everyone else. Must demographics somehow be twisted to suffice, or can we tweak the system? Can we all live ninety years, and only work for thirty of them?

The Demographic Distribution of Health Costs. Unfortunately, health costs do not self-distribute to match health revenues without some pushing. Mostly, the process is, revenues are twisted to match costs.

About 3% of health costs concentrate in the first year of life, about 15% of costs are generated in the last year of life. The last year of life itself has shifted, from age 47 in 1900 to 83, today. Given some time, longevity will grow to 93. From these facts alone we see a minimum of 18% of costs being redistributed from workers to non-workers, and inter-generational cost shifts as a whole are probably closer to 68%. That's variable and inaccurate, because hospitals know you have to be born and you have to die, so they find ways to pad bills, shifting the cost of what isn't mandatory, onto the bills of those who cannot escape. That in turn is shifted a second time, to the people who can better afford to pay them. It seem to the business office like money going in

> *"Mostly, revenues are twisted to match costs."*
> **Hospital Cost Shifting**

and out of the accounting office door, but in fact it goes in one door, and goes out through quite a different door.

63

It just has to be that way; no other way will work. It isn't rocket science to figure out, it actually doesn't cost thousands of dollars to deliver a baby, or to pronounce an old fellow dead. Just compare the price of a five-star hotel with the price of (one half of) a semiprivate hospital room, or the cost of a frozen food dinner with a hospital meal. This isn't cheating; it's just an institution trying to serve the community.

Indirect Overhead. One of the generalizations which is made fairly, however, is a typical hospital ends up with too much indirect overhead. Somebody has to be paid to mow the lawn, but you can't very well bill patients individually for lawn-cutting. Somebody must answer the telephone for the institution. Over the past centuries, a lot of activity was dumped on the hospital, because hospitals are nice, they are handy, and everybody shares a piece. They are a favorite place to hold local elections on the second Tuesday in November, for example, because they generally have some spare space in the lobby, and they belong to everybody in the community. They have cafeterias and gift shops because that is part of their function. As long as they have them, why can't the community use them? They also have parking garages, partly with the same motive banks use, to issue mortgages for buildings which could be sold for some other use in a pinch. And mortgages are cheap, right now. The point is not they are building things they don't really need, the point is an accumulation of such costs provides a handy vehicle for – large indirect overhead charges on the cost report. Every overhead cost must eventually be added to some bill, and can thus – why not – be re-assigned to areas of the hospital which normally house patients of a target group.

There once was a time when indirect costs avoided elderly patients; as soon as Medicare became an entitlement, the incentives shifted. Now, serious expensive diseases are all migrating into the Medicare age group. As they do with computerized cost-shifting of pediatric units, and as they will when Obamacare pays for some indigents. But please don't pass regulations to suppress the salaries of cost accountants, in order to control all this abuse you have suddenly discovered.

When 100% of the costs must be supported by 20% of the patients, no hospital in existence could stay in business for a week, without cost-shifting. No doubt, most hospital administrators would welcome insurance companies doing this cost-shifting on their own books, but they would be foolish to permit it. Sooner or later, some community activist would protest it was dishonest, and the insurance companies would promptly dump it back in the hospitals' laps. In a sense, hospitals are reinsurers of last resort, and must remain reluctant to give away the tools of their trade.

Diagnosis Related Groups (DRG), in Relation to Medical Electronic Records.

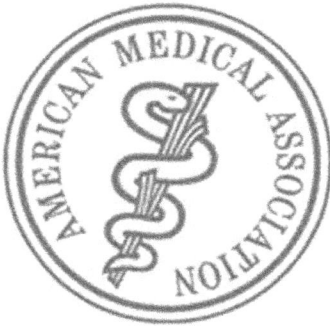

The American Medical Association

For a concept supposedly working moderately well, the Diagnosis Related Groups (DRG) system for inpatient reimbursement has a bizarre history. It has led to some unconfessed, and widely unrecognized, disastrous results, and should be thoroughly reworked as soon as possible. In a scholarly sense, the story begins eighty years ago. The American Medical Association decided all of disease, ultimately all of medical care, would be better understood if reduced to a systematized code. Originally, the code was visualized as a six digit complex, with the first three digits defining anatomical location, followed by a second set of three digits specifying the cause of the disease affecting that location.

SNODO That 6-digit structure limited a code to a thousand diseases in a thousand locations, or a million "disorders" just for a beginning. Roughly half those theoretical combinations have no biologic existence, although even fanciful codes had some value for detecting coding errors. Other regions of the code exceeded the number of conditions actually found to exist, but originating in a digital structure then allowed virtually unlimited expansion, but sacrificed the significance of a particular position within the code. IBM was enlisted as a consultant, who advised the AMA to stop worrying about it; just provide a numerical code for everything, in the finest detail possible. Mathematicians could later easily make it usable for calculating machines, the forerunners of computers; and non-existent conditions created no harm. Some of those consultants had worked with a system which produced great success for the U.S. Census, and perceived no advantage to limiting the code numbers, while planning for them to be manipulated by machines. A third group of three digits was soon added, making a nine-digit *Standard Nomenclature of Diseases and Operations*, familiarly known as SNODO, which could identify a million different operations, whether actually performed or not. Actually, groups of three or more digits separated into groups of three digits by hyphens, transferred the significance of code-position to the cluster level, which proved adequate.

SNOMED The pathology profession subsequently added still a fourth set of digits, for microscopic features, so the potential was soon up to a hundred million microscopic conditions. The team of physicians who worked on coding the medical universe contains many names now famous, notably including Robert F. Loeb and Dana Atchley of The College of Physicians and Surgeons of Columbia University. For at least thirty years, the Joint Commission on the Accreditation of Hospitals (an AMA and AHA joint affiliate) enforced a rule: every discharge summary from every accredited hospital in America must code and index every discharge diagnosis in SNODO code. It was tedious work, kept alive by the glittering future prospect of developing an Electronic Medical Record by 1940.

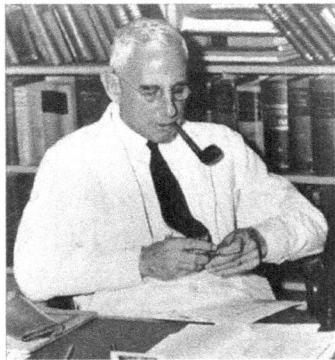

Robert F. Loeb

ICDA After twenty years or so of this enormous task, the Medical Records Librarians rebelled. The labor effort was burdensome, and the librarians were in an occupational position to observe how little use was being made of it. On their demand, an alternative simpler coding system was adopted, called the *International Classification of Diseases (ICDA)*. At first it was limited to the one thousand commonest discharge diagnoses, therefore limited to the charts which the librarians could confidently observe would be used. In time, it was expanded to ten thousand commonest diagnoses. Limiting medical codes also limited the cost and effort of coding, and was considered an important retreat from over-enthusiasm. Meanwhile, expansion of the SNODO code by a handful of true believers continued to fill up the coding gaps, soon using and exceeding the capacity of the 80-column IBM punch card (originally, ten digits plus metadata), one card per diagnosis.

Unfortunately, the code was in danger of collapsing from this unanticipated expansion, since computers had not yet advanced to the point where they could rescue SNODO from the limitations apparent to its users. It was a classic case of a hypothetical system appearing to be better than the one in actual use, but not living up to its promise when both systems encountered actual use. The ICDA coding scheme did suffice for immediate purposes, and the "calculator" system was at least a decade away from evolving into the more flexible "computer" which could skip around the limitations of a punched card input system.

The professional difference was this: the doctors roughly understood the coding logic, and could devise an understandable code for most charts through the logic of a structured language. The record librarians had not been trained to encipher (or even dither, as photographers say) the code by logic; a thousand codes was about the limit of what anyone could memorize. The burden of manual coding eventually overran the code design, before practical results could defend its utility in other areas of the hospital or the profession.

All the medical record world promptly abandoned SNODO; except for the pathologists who intuitively recognized ICDA could never approach their own greatly expanded needs. Eventually pathologists took SDODO over, expanded and redesigned the basic framework, and produced what they are rightly proud of, an elegant code book called SNOmed which obeyed meaningful internal coding rules. It still came however, as a large and expensive book, which most practitioners were reluctant either to buy, or to use.

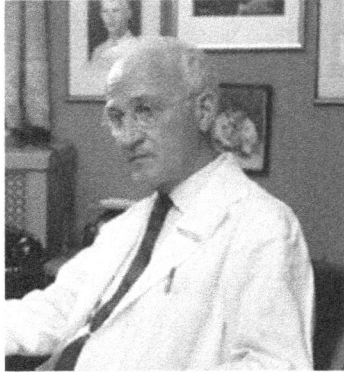

Dana Atchley

DRG Meanwhile, a group at the School of Hospital Administration at Yale under the leadership of John Thompson lurched in the opposite direction of drastically reducing the ICDA code (initially expanded to 10,000 entries, which proved too large for some purposes, while still lacking specificity in many others), back down to only 468 of the commonest "diagnosis clusters". The purpose was to find clusters of diagnoses with common characteristics, which could be used by unskilled employees to identify diagnosis submissions which normally fell within certain bounds, but who in a particular case were sufficiently deviant to warrant investigation as "outriders". This gross sorting by machine was then examined by the PSRO (Professional Standards Review Organizations), especially in the central feature of length of stay. They termed their product *Diagnosis-Related Groups (DRG)*, which made no pretense of being complete, but was complete enough to encompass the majority of outrider events. The computer version of their concept was called Autogrp, which had some attraction to hospital administrations as a way to predict outriders. To summarize what happened next when Medicare adopted DRG for payment purposes: both DRG and ICDA started to expand, and

> *"Two million diagnoses are compressed into two hundred payment groups."*
> **Diagnosis "Related" Groups**

68

SNOMED was relegated to the role of code book for Neanderthal pathologists.

Using the standard diagnosis codes, one- size-fits-all did not help the hospital and insurance accountants a bit, since by habit they tend to believe all businesses are about the same, no matter what the business produces. Their complaint was codes with thousands of codes were too big and complicated. Simultaneously the medical professionals were finding them much too small for the job. Meanwhile, ICDA was fast losing its reputation for being compact and inexpensive, while the opposite feeling immediately developed: the DRG was far too small for what physicians could now realize was going to play a very large and important role in everybody's finances. Two vital areas of the hospital had difficulty communicating from the beginning; now, there was no longer even a common language to use. There was no quick fix, either, because both DRG and the underlying ICDA designs were based on frequency of occurrence, rather than precision and logic. Furthermore, the copyright was owned by professional societies who had little interest in finances, and considerable interest in reducing their burdensome coding workload. In the background, however, computers had made the task of code translation a trivial one. A third profession, the computer department, scarcely knew what the other two were talking about, but they came closer to affinity with the accountants.

Like the three bears of Goldilocks, some codes were too large and some were too small, but at least there were three of them, each crippled in a different way. Comparatively few doctors understood what was going on, and in spite of their vital interest at stake, had trouble getting over their hatred of the boring coding task. Since this whole issue of data coding and summarization has taken on major importance to the success of the Affordable Care Act, in some circles the uproar has become a political war dance. Let Obama do it, if he likes coding so much. Basically, the librarians were saying they resented being criticized for making important mistakes in a task they didn't understand very well. In summary, everybody hates coding.

Overview of the Future. One faction of the small field of those who are interested in such matters, has decided to expand both the specificity and the reach of ICDA, which is now up to its tenth edition of revision. Unfortunately, it does not seem to some of the pathologists to be a sensible approach. We have an elegant code in SNOMED, they protested, which is arguably too big to use; expanding ICDA seems destined to reach the same destination, on the rebound from being too small. We now have ample data on what is common. The most efficient approach would at first seem to be condensing the highly specific SNOMED to a useful size, based on frequency of use. The approach would stand in contrast to making a list of diseases by frequency, and then subdividing their specificities. While such a condensed volume could be printed as a book, we are now at a point where every record room within the hospitals of the nation is equipped with several computers, so elasticity of the code should no longer be anyone's problem. Let the machines do the drudgery.

This whole process could now rather easily be automated for much more than its original purpose of classifying disease populations, and in a pinch it could even substitute 26-digit letters for 10-digit numerals, imparting some clues in the process. A further condensation of an already condensed version began to be used for payment purposes, adding still greater amounts of practical nuance. You might suppose everyone could see paying the same amount of money for treating the same disease (tuberculosis, let's say) of two different organs (let's say of bone, and of kidney) was either going to bankrupt someone, or enrich someone else. And that's only money. Any scientific or diagnostic decision based on a code of "All other" will make computerized medical records sprint faster toward worthlessness. At the rate it's going, lumps of "all other" will have no relation to each other, except to justify the same reimbursement for treatments of vastly different value. Or difficulty. Or cost. Or contagiousness.

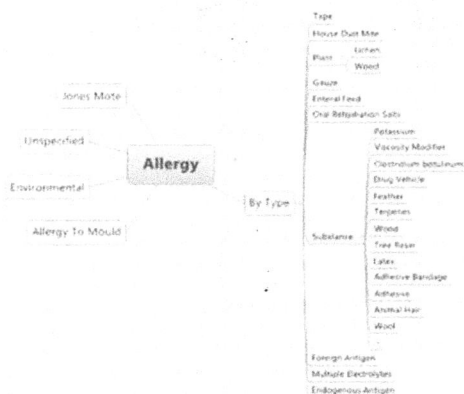

Tape
House Dust Mite
Lichen
Plant
Wood
Gauze
Enteral Feed
Oral Rehydration Salts
Potassium
Viscosity Modifier
Clostridium botulinum
Drug Vehicle
Feather
Terpenes
Wood
Tree Rosin
Latex
Adhesive Bandage
Adhesive
Animal Hair
Wool
Foreign Antigen
Multiple Electrolytes
Endogenous Antigen

Jones Mote
Unspecified
Allergy
Environmental
By Type
Allergy to Mould
Substance

SNOMED

In automated form, SNOMED is quite ready to be revised still further in other directions for other purposes. It could, for once, integrate the accounting and demographic functions with the rest of medical care. But a great many other useful functions can be imagined, once computers have a stable platform on which to build, and the task of coding can be safely undertaken without much physician input burden. Safe, that is, from the danger the whole coding framework will get changed, again and again. In a certain sense, this is similar to the brilliant choice by Apple of the Unix skeleton, when Microsoft Windows seized on quicker expedients. A great many sub-professions seem to wish to have their own codes for their own purposes, and resist the idea a physician code should be imposed on them. When you encounter such obstructionism, it is easy to suspect motives. But the general rule is: when it comes to a choice between scheming and incompetence, it's incompetence, nine times out of ten.

However, medical care and hospital care are medical functions, and their accounting and demographics will always eventually return to their medical professional core. Meanwhile, notice what happened to DRG, a code so crude it relegates most refinements to the category of "All Other". The fact of the matter is, it is a crude approximation, some cases paying on the high side, some on the low side of true costs. If the hospital loses money on inpatients, well, just build another wing to the outpatient department. Underlying this response was the enduring misconception that outpatient care is inherently cheaper than inpatient. If it's the case, well, we'll just have to fix it.

The surprising lack of chaos from such expedience has almost nothing to do with medical content, and almost everything to do with having insufficient case volume to remain in balance. That is, the big hospitals smudge it out, and the small hospitals don't understand it. The highly prized profit margin of 2% or 3% can easily be achieved by admitting slightly more cases of a profitable kind (ie hire a surgeon expert in certain profitable operations), or by the government adjusting just a few DRGs to profitable status (like reducing tariffs on behalf of favored industries in Congress). Meanwhile, the rest of the enterprise becomes progressively more expensive, because there is no fixed relationship between service benefit prices and audited costs, and now an even less regular relation, to cost-to-charge ratios.

It is a precarious thing for institutional solvency, to depend on financial balancing of a particular case load within one set of four walls, and then complain hospitals are too small to survive. Between their accountants and their record librarians, this outcome drives the smaller institution into a futile chase after higher patient volume. Of course we need to change with the times. But some basic truths never change, and one of them is every ship should be able to sail on its own bottom. You don't approach that by giving every ship a new hull.

Let's get specific. In the first place, allowing only a 2% profit margin during a 3% national inflation is to walk on the edge of a dangerous cliff. If some fair profit margin could be agreed to, it is only an average among hospitals. You might as well reduce the DRG to four payment levels, and reimburse hospitals on the basis of which of the four walls the patient faces. With enough tinkering, you might arrive at the desired total hospital reimbursement to match any profit margin you establish, totally disregarding the diagnoses of all patients. Quite obviously, you must code the diagnosis to whatever number of digits it requires to identify the unique condition. You could match up all of the hundred dollar cases and all of the fifty thousand dollar cases, call the two codes, and pay only two prices.

But such an effort is just a delusion. Somebody – or some machine – has to go to the trouble of coding every single diagnosis down to the point where the code is no longer meaningful to costs, and assign relative values among them. Only at that point would it be legitimate to assign a dollar amount to each relative value. You have to maintain the code as treatments change, which will be quite frequently. You can do it, and you can computerize it. A computerized version of this process would scarcely be any different from copying the English description and, like a Google search, getting back a number to copy; it might even be done by voice transcription. But there is still no guarantee charging itemized bills wouldn't turn out to be cheaper, and at least have a different meaning. DRG in its present form is nothing but a crude rationing system; get rid of it, or spend the money to make it work. I can't guarantee if you put a doctor in charge, it would work. But I can guarantee that if you don't put a doctor in charge, it won't.

> **Proposal 5:** Congress should be asked to commission a computer program to translate English language diagnoses into SNOMED code, preferably by voice translation. Suggested format: a search engine where English variants of discharge diagnoses are entered, and a SNOMED code number returned, along the general lines of entering common phrases into Google and receiving file location numbers in return, except it returns the SNOMED code. If the code is not found, the computer accepts a manual entry by a trained person. verified by an expert over the Internet to become officially entered into a master list which is periodically circulated as an update. The search program and its supplements should be produced on DVD disks to be used on hospital record room computers by other professional users. It should provide "hooks" so the Snomed codes and patient identification can be transferred electronically to related programs, such as payment codes and billing.

So that's how DRG got to be what it is. It's perfectly astounding such a crudity, devised for other purposes, could be so "successfully" employed to pay for billions of dollars of Medicare inpatient care, such that payment by diagnosis-lumps threatens to spread to all medical care. There is even another way to describe it: inpatient hospital care has been lumped into a rationing system which constrains national inpatient care to a 2% overall average profit margin. That's just as surely true as if someone deliberately tried to make it that way.

Payment by diagnosis ignores both cost and content, based on the mistaken assumption those features have already been carefully accounted for. It does not matter in the slightest how long the patient stays or how many tests he gets, or how many expensive big hospitals swallow up inexpensive little ones. Meanwhile, emergency rooms and satellite clinics also do not affect the cost inherent in a supposed linkage between the diagnosis and the cost. The failure to link drug prices into this modified market system, is particularly noticeable.

The exciting potential has been lost to have the patients who can shop frugally as outpatients, set the price for inpatients who are helpless to act frugally. Their much more generous profit margins support what is essentially a hospital conglomerate. Any corporate conglomerate executive could tell you what happens when one department is subsidized, while another is treated as a cash cow. And the fun part is this: squeezing physician income against an unsustainable "Sustainable" Growth Rate creates the "doc fix", which annually blackmails physicians into acquiescence past the next November elections.

SGR: Sustainable growth rate, earmarks by a different name. SGR is a term borrowed from financial economics, signifying the rate at which a company is able to grow without borrowing more money. It is easily calculated by subtracting dividends from return on investment. Any variation from this definition, will produce different results. A sustainable growth rate in Medicare is calculated by a formula, modified every year in special ways which closely resemble "earmarks", but contain special adjustments for changing work hour components, malpractice cost components, etc. It is a large task for the Physician Payment Commission to determine yearly changes in thousands of services, and it must be frustrating for them to see their painstaking calculations tossed aside every year by Congress, in response to howls from the various professions. Whenever this occurs it is a fair guess the calculation has been misused. The discussion has long since transformed from a simple calculation to a simple threat: physician reimbursement will be cut. Each year it is cut, and each year Congress relents on the cut at the last moment. But ultimately its design will prevail: on the pie-chart of healthcare expense, physician reimbursement will shrink, and hospital reimbursement will expand, as physicians migrate to salaried hospital employment, and enjoy an instant 40-hour week amidst a physician shortage. This keeps the AMA in a constant state of agitation, and physicians in a constant posture of supplication. At the end of 2013, the proposed cut in reimbursement had grown to 26%. When almost every physician has an overhead of 50%, a cut of 26% is beyond meaningful. And every year the financial attractiveness of joining a hospital clinic for a dependable salary grows, with consequent improvement in overall power of the hospital conglomerate, and steadily decreasing relation to market-set pricing readjustments.

Insurance Reimbursement, The Missing Item on the Itemized Bill. The DRG system threatens patients, too. After discharge from a hospital, the patient is sent a multi-page itemized bill, which purports to be what the patient would owe without insurance. Such bills traditionally omit any mention of the insurance reimbursement, which is the only payment the hospital receives if it has contracted to accept "service benefits" as payment in full. Since that is almost always the case, the "total of service benefits" is exactly equal to the "total patient responsibility". Since the patient will pay nothing if patient responsibility is limited to service benefits, and service benefits are exactly equal to whatever the patient received, the explanation goes round and round without ever revealing what has been paid. The illusion that you have been told something worth hearing, is maintained by providing an almost endless list of itemized charges.

Most hospital employees do not have the foggiest idea why the list is even produced, and its accuracy is therefore questionable. A variety of specious explanations therefore emerge, usually with a focus on billing a handful of uninsured people, or insured people whose service benefits have expired as "outriders". There may be a particle of truth to this, easily refuted by showing the supposed items on the bill were often fabricated by employees who know very well they are seldom used for anything. Most likely, the purpose is to conceal the true insurance reimbursement from competitive insurances who might undercut them. As profit margins shrink, it becomes increasingly dangerous to let competitors know what they are. As margins widen, it is even easier for competitors to undercut them. As a matter of common observation, most retailers in any business are less than forthright about their profit margins, so perhaps this concealment can be forgiven as normal commercial behavior. It becomes more questionable when seen as an industry-wide practice, intended to defend a system of double-pricing. In this case, it defends the employer tax discount as the lowest price around, when compared with those rascals, the uninsured or the insured but fully taxed.

The DRG payment to the hospital is not zero, but it is far less than the total on the itemized bill, and is seldom revealed. One central message it sends is however pretty clear: "This is how much you would be charged, if you didn't have Insurance X." The shortfall in revenue is made up by overcharging the emergency room and the outpatients, who are unsuitable for anything resembling the present DRG. If the hospital does not have enough outpatient work to sustain the inpatient losses, its only recourse at present is to call the architects and build a bigger outpatient department. To fill it, just buy up a neighboring group practice or two of neighborhood doctors. Fix the DRG, and it would be hard to say what would eventuate.

Bottom Line: Who is Injured? For a long time, service benefit insurance was the only thing supporting the hospital industry, and commercial behavior by the hospitals was justified as the only way to support their charitable mission. Now that Health Savings Accounts have reached 12 million clients, with assets reaching $22.8 billion, a viable way to provide indemnity insurance has definitely arrived. Not only are HSAs cheaper for the customer, they very likely provide higher payments to hospitals. This last point will only be clarified when we learn what discounts the catastrophic high-deductible insurance have been able to extract, but hardly anything else will affect the answer. To the extent one competitive method receives major discounts and the others generally do not, this service benefit discount is probably only of benefit to the insurance companies who enjoy it. A personal episode in my family illustrates.

My son went to a well-known Boston hospital for an outpatient colonoscopy, and received a bill for $8000.00. When told that was outrageous, he protested and promptly received a bill reducing the charge to $1000. He was delighted to send a check for that reduced amount, even though I told him a fair price was probably around $300. He reminded me of a comment from a famous surgeon now deceased, whose name is emblazoned on a tall pavilion in another city. The old surgeon growled, "The only reason to carry health insurance is to keep the hospital from fleecing you." In a sense, that growl applied directly to the colonoscopy, which that hospital had converted from a markup into a holdup.

Discounts for Health Savings Accounts? HSAs scarcely have to penetrate the market much further before they have the market power to command an equal discount. That may still take a little time, because some states have hardly any penetration, while California has a million subscribers. In the meantime, the patient needs to be careful to ask for prices in advance. Almost every health insurance has started to impose high deductibles, so their proper stance is to insist on equal treatment. The old system of "First-dollar coverage" was responsible for making outpatient care a target for this sort of thing. The next advance, after making all outpatient care match market prices, is to insist a hospital charge the same thing for the same service for inpatients as it does with outpatients. To make that possible, it has to return to fee-for-service billing, and managements of Health Savings Accounts should settle for no less. That's the main reason DRG billing offends me, although there are lots of other reasons, and lots of other people are injured in different ways.

Hospital Cost-Shifting Reacts to the DRG

Medicare's payment-by-diagnosis system requires a diagnosis code for its computers to specify the payment. Codes are the way doctors can conduct their activities on a medical level, while revealing to the billing department what the activity is worth. The billing department knows well enough these values will be later smudged and bloated, so why make work for yourself being accurate? Careful, fellows, your foot is on a slippery path.

High-handed Codes. The government could have chosen a coding system called SnoMed (Standard Nomenclature of Medicine), which specifies several million diagnoses in detail. Or it could have specified ICDA (International Classification of Diseases), which in its various iterations can identify several thousand. What it did choose was DRG, or Diagnosis-related Groups, specifying about two hundred. With various adjustments and offsets, this translates: there are only two hundred different price buttons to push – for millions of diagnoses. The theory is, some cases will cost more, some will cost less, but in the long run it all comes out just exactly right. Saves work for the billing clerks, that way.

Careful, fellows, you have stepped over the line of what is allowable latitude. Buried in your computer cubicles, hidden behind green eyeshades, you have convinced yourselves the world will tolerate anything you do for your own convenience. Try talking to one of them some time – you will surely find the door is locked, or the boss is out to lunch, or it isn't company policy to allow accountants to talk to outsiders. If you have credentials, you may talk to a spokesman who seems to keep repeating himself. It does not seem to have occurred to anyone that the public wants to know if the charges are fair, and at the very least has a right to know if they are accurate. How can they be either fair or accurate, if millions of activities are reduced to two hundred price buttons?

> *"Pure and simple:*
> *A rationing system."*
> **DRG**

I remember well, sitting in the Congressional hearing room when this proposal was first made. I giggled over Congress letting someone even utter such nonsense, let alone pass a law to go ahead with using it. But now I have to listen to reports this system has been in place for twenty years, and it works just wonderfully fine. A friend of mine was a graduate student at Yale, helping to develop the DRG system in its original form. He, too, is appalled that such an unexpected usage could even be considered, for what had an entirely different original purpose. The DRG was part of a coding system devised to assist the Professional Standards Review Organizations in monitoring insurance claims for errors and fraud. The behavior of each diagnosis group was studied for its general outline, and general patterns were identified. If a case fell outside the norms, it was tagged for investigation. Just how well DRG's worked out for that particular purpose, I have no idea. But to extend it for actual payment of particular claims, simply boggled the mind, and still does.

Children Playing With Matches. When you let people do things like that, some pretty unexpected things happen. In the first place, using a system tailor-made for Medicare, you need at least one extra system to pay for patients who don't have Medicare. However, Medicare accounts for about half of average hospital revenue, so there is automatic pressure on everybody to conform to the system of the big cajuna. An elaborate system called Chargemaster was devised for itemized services to be listed on an itemized bill, which now runs to dozens of pages for each patient. Since nobody much was going to use anything but DRG, the reasoning went that constant revision of thousands of itemized charges would be a big and useless task. Since you had to do it, you set the charges so high you wouldn't have to come back and revise them so often. Countless reporters have asked dozens of hospital administrators to explain the itemized bills which emerge, and almost every administrator admits he doesn't understand Chargemaster, and never looks at it.

Chargemaster. The billing clerks of the hospital look at it, however, and the patients look, and reporters look. Itemized bills totalling tens of thousands of dollars are sent, first to the patients, and then to the bill collectors. Stephen Brill's *America's Bitter Pill* is filled with "Tom and Mary of Tuscon" anecdotes, so let me add a couple of personal ones. For example, I received a bill for Seven thousand dollars from my own hospital accident room for twenty minutes treatment for a sprained wrist; the hospital clerk had joined in such a welcoming reunion for old times' sake, he forgot to collect my insurance numbers. After several strikingly threatening letters, communication eventually stopped. I have to assume they eventually found my insurance numbers on the record of an earlier admission. In another case, I discovered that another of my hospitals sends its bills when tests are ordered, not when they are performed. Consequently, a patient I discharged from the accident room without having the tests the interne had ordered, received an astonishing bill for the services, anyway. Since he was vice-president of the insurance company which covered him, there were some gratifying repercussions. On a later occasion, my oldest son received a bill for $8,500 for a colonoscopy from a famous Boston Hospital, and asked me what I thought was fair. I said it was worth a couple hundred dollars, so he called his insurance company, following which the revised bill was one thousand dollars. He fell all over himself writing a check, for what I still say was a gross overcharge. Notice one theme running through all of these true stories. *They all involved outpatient services.*

You see, the hospitals were all shifting to a Chargemaster system for outpatients, because the inpatient charges (often for the same services) were frozen by the DRG. In fact, it is widely quoted that inpatient profit margins were 2%, accident room profit margins were 15%, and the outpatient area made a profit of 30%. If anything approaching that

> *"If you put physicians on salaries, you get an instant forty-hour week. Soon, you get physician shortages."*

is true, well, what would you do in their place? The next time you go past your local hospital, try to notice if a construction crane is working on a new building. The chances are excellent you will find it's a new outpatient building.

After all, with the Federal Reserve promoting the zero interest boundary, mortgages are pretty cheap. Right now is an excellent time to build a building, if you ever think you might need one. So, some of these buildings might be designed to house group practices. If a hospital plans to go into the outpatient business, it needs a lot of doctors. A shrinking minority of physicians are still in private practice, so it's getting hard to find a doctor. Hospital-salaried physicians are easy to hire, but hard to get on the telephone, and even harder to find on nights and weekends. If you put physicians on salaries, you will get an almost instant forty-hour week. As the husband, father, and nephew of female physicians, it is a little unbecoming of me to observe that a majority of medical students are women these days, and of course it delights the feminists. But it's also true that women physicians have a biologic need for regular hours, retire earlier, and seek out specialties which accommodate them. Women like to be in groups, because there are fewer times to be on call for holidays and weekends which you can share more widely. You will need more women physicians to do the same job that men do, so the public can eventually expect higher costs for the same service. By the way, with three women physicians in my immediate family, I never once heard a complaint from them about male discrimination.

Hospitals are busy buying up physician practices because of the indirect effect of the DRG. Furthermore, the prices are high and the government is paying the bill through the hospital reimbursement system. My old friends smile, and wink they will go back into practice if the hospital reimbursement declines. That long-term cost has to be factored in, although I doubt it will happen as they age. But if it does, the cost of reconciling a physician surplus might have to be included in the eventual reckoning of what the DRG did or did not save.

When you get down to it, the DRG is an excellent rationing tool, and rationing invariably creates shortages. Robert Morris learned that lesson the hard way during the Revolutionary War. He didn't speak much during the Constitutional Convention in 1789, but he was utterly determined that we not construct a command economy – which is rationing on a grander scale. He kept his attention on his own business, while his protégé Alexander Hamilton did the talking, and his best friend George Washington did the listening. How is the DRG a rationing tool? The government makes the rules, sets the prices, and monitors the outcome. However you choose to achieve a 2% inpatient profit margin, its economic effect is remorselessly judged as 2% revenue, operating within a 2% inflation rate, achieved by a 2% inflation target at the Federal Reserve. All the slack in the system has seemingly been driven into the out-patient and accident room areas. Except it hasn't. Everything the inpatient system asks for, shall be given to it, on a 2% cost-plus basis. Profit margin, indeed. What we have is a cost-plus procurement system.

The Doc Fix

Unless a Congressman's name is attached to it by the media, it generally isn't easy to know who was the originator of a disagreeable law. In the case of Medicare, moreover, the program is technically an amendment to the Social Security Act, so revenue amendments must originate in the House of Representatives, Committee on Ways and Means, Subcommittee on Health. The difficulty is easily fixed by the Senate making an amendment to some unrelated House bill such as housing relief in Kansas. All subsequent amendments must jump through the same hoops, because Congress is very strict about such traditions.

At any rate, some amendment was passed by both Houses to the effect that doctors' reimbursement would be held down if general Medicare costs had risen more than a certain amount. The theory was of course that doctors are in control of all medical costs, and therefore should be punished if they rose too high. The real purpose was to keep the doctors docile and quiet, since at the last moment, each and every year, an exception to the punishment was made, just for one more year. This went on for eighteen years, until Republicans finally achieved a majority in both Houses of Congress, and the law was promptly repealed in 2014. It was now possible to be pretty sure who had been behind the law all along. To reinforce this identification, the Senate Majority leader, Mitch McConnell (R, Ky.) executed a flashy last-minute parliamentary maneuver to rescue the repeal from its unidentified enemies, who had surely been of the other party. The "doc fix" was finally fixed.

In the course of this wrangle, it was revealed that physicians received 12% of Medicare expenditures. It reminded me, I had published a graph in *The Hospital That Ate Chicago*, showing that physicians received 20% in 1980. That would suggest their reimbursement had fallen by 8%, and perhaps that is true, corrected for inflation. However, reimbursements to other providers have risen, so the net change in physician reimbursement might be different from 8%. However, a related but different factor probably played an important part in this shift. Also during that period, a majority of physicians changed from solo private practice to working on a salary provided by a hospital group practice. The net effect was to shift the spokesmen for doctors' financial interests. It used to be the American Medical Association, and now was to be hospital administration. In time, substance will follow form.

True, the primary cause of this shift was DRG pressure to shift revenue to the outpatient area, but since hospitals also participate in the Henry Kaiser tax dodge, this incentive was also at work, in a combined or concerted effect. The overall reimbursement effect was to shift physician overhead out of the costs, but not out of the reimbursement, which now goes to the hospital. Since almost every physician in practice spends 50% of his gross revenue on office overhead, there is plenty of room for shifts which do not appear on the balance sheet. Yes, physicians temporarily protected their net income by this maneuver, but the hospitals acquired an expense they did not necessarily intend to maintain. Squeeze the hospitals with DRG or other means, and politicians as well as hospitals had a piggy bank they could always return to, in a pinch.

The Doc fix has finally been repealed, possibly in part because it has served its several purposes. But tickling the victim for campaign contributions hasn't been repealed. This ancient parliamentary maneuver is unaffected. It will return, in other guises.

Reverse Bribery. Still another seemingly tangential issue is in the news, six months after control of Congress shifted parties. An ordinary layman would wonder if a 2.5% tax on medical devices is worth the acrimony its repeal seems to engender. But the ordinary layman is not familiar with bare-knuckle Chicago politics. When the Affordable Care Act was approaching legislative action, most of the affected groups were approached to sign up. Behind the enticements was an unspoken threat: if you don't come on board, you will be sorry. With only one notable exception (the medical device people), everyone signed on. And then the 2.5% special tax was laid on Medical devices. If you wonder why such small matters stir up so much bitterness, the history of the legislative preliminaries would seem of value to the search.

Amending Laws Rather than Rejecting Them

Dision of power is one of the strengths of our system of governance. Isolating power to authorize spending, from power to spend, serves as an example. It's rather different, if one side seems to be winning all the battles; some fundamental power should possibly then be shifted. If the Founders believed God wound up the Universe clock and then let it run by itself, it seemed sensible to organize all government operations the same way. Entropy does not pick political favorites.

Very likely, the founders underestimated the time it would take for final balance to be struck between these two viewpoints, because it is nearly always the majority opinion which needs to be resisted. That's the unwritten assumption about what today is called Quaker Process, which occasionally irritates jumpy people. But nevertheless, in two hundred years, only slavery has seemed intractably unbalanced enough to warrant re-balancing by force. The Supreme Court-packing episode of 1937 came pretty close, ultimately shifting commerce regulation from states to federal. But it should have been done by amendment. Deleting the word "interstate" from the "interstate commerce" clause, must have seemed clever. That innovative way of amending the Constitution by one-word amendment has now lasted nearly a century, has never been exactly repeated, and surely would be reversed if the states could discover a way to regain their intended former power. Parsimony of words is admirable, but to have Courts amending the substance of a law is not in the province of either the Judicial or Executive branch. It takes some process the minority will agree to.

The Roberts Court seems to be continuing the "interstate" example of reversing policy by shifting the meaning of substantive words, as in "tax" and "penalty", when almost everyone agrees more orthodox amendment is more civil. Revising the meaning of "State exchanges" to include "Federal exchanges", clearly exceeds public tolerance for unorthodox approaches to language, however. If that's where they are going, the Court better slow down before their example is taken by lower courts, and ultimately by common practice. If you want to be treated like a leader, you must act like one. Our doctors in 1965, if not our lawmakers, had noticed Canada offering block grants to provinces who adopted the National Health system, which even Quebec felt forced to accept if they were going to be taxed for it, anyway. It seems particularly

> *"The Interstate Commerce Clause became the Commerce Clause, and Penalties became Taxes."*
> **THE LIVING CONSTITUTION**

extortionate when applied to the Affordable Care Act. Our Supreme Court was primarily declaring, hinted extortion of this sort was unacceptable because of repeated Executive Branch examples of it.

That a majority of the Court was willing to reverse the meaning of language even after previously striking federal coercion in the same law, probably reflects the underlying opinion of one wavering Justice rather than the whole Court, while the Chief Justice struggled to maintain authorship of the decision. In the long view, elections rather than a few altered words may clarify the legal point. But an opportunity has been created for opportunists to move faster than the whole Court usually would.

In the case of *King v. Burwell* much the same thing as in the Court-packing episode happened, but in a law rather than the Constitution. Just as the word "Interstate" was deleted to read "Commerce Clause", while in the other, "State and Federal Exchanges" became "exchanges". The original language of the Act, about who can extend subsidies, was reversed to mean its opposite. This additionally has the subtle effect of endorsing the Legislative practice, demonstrated in this legislation, of placing deliberately opposite views into House and Senate versions, in order to conceal the real intention until the conference committee meets, the press is absent, and a holiday is near. In this case, it has the alternative appearance to the public that some members of the Court may have been better informed about the facts behind drafting the bill, than others.

A cloud of conflicting stories were printed after the decision, and it is hard to judge which one was truthful. My own preference is for the book by Jacob S. Hacker, *The Road to Nowhere*, written from interviews years earlier about the maneuvers of Hillary Clinton's allies for the Clinton Health Plan. Hacker now sounds particularly pertinent, since he was active in the Obama campaign, and because the reasoning of the majority about "ambiguity" sounds so strained. The suspicion of cover stories is regrettable. The public likes to believe the cloistered Supreme Court *does not* read the newspapers, as Mr. Dooley once put it, and only acts on testimony under oath in front of opposing counsel. That may be physically impossible, but the appearance is worth preserving.

Methods in the Madness

E ven today, many people are uncomfortable about psychiatric illness in their family. In the Nineteenth century, this feeling was much more pronounced, so wealthy families sought out luxurious psychiatric hospitals where wealthy patients were kept out of sight. Rich families also sought out psychiatrists of their own class to be in charge; not only keeping matters out of sight, they were also likely to be discreet in their outside discussions. Sigmund Freud wrote a whole book to the effect that getting richer brings on mental disorders.

Snake Pits. By contrast, saying institutions for indigent psychiatric patients were once substandard, is quite an understatement. Indigent cost to society must have been a considerable burden fifty years ago, with over 500,000 licensed beds nationally in 1955, even though society is a notorious pinch-penny with indigents in any era. When Thorazine made its appearance as the first really effective anti-psychotic drug in 1953, it was prematurely followed in 1955 by President Kennedy announcing a plan for cutting the number of inpatient psychiatric beds by half. This goal was quickly and drastically achieved, cutting beds in "psychiatric snake-pits" to 40,000 by year 2000. To a certain degree, however, we have simply moved mental patients from snake pits into prisons at higher cost. In all this turmoil, upper-class institutions at first were much less affected.

Rest Cures. During the last half of the Nineteenth century, psychiatry itself had become a distinctly upper-class specialty. To what extent this class isolation was a cause of the profession's later troubles is hard to say, but it probably was a factor. In the early Twentieth century, this social situation was upset by a pell-mell rush of enthusiasm by psychiatrists to follow the teachings of the Austrian doctor, Sigmund Freud, introducing psychoanalytic methods of treatment at significantly higher cost.

The Analysts. For a while, no academic psychiatrist could expect promotion unless he was an analyst, and this attitude spread out into the practicing profession, too. But its time was brief; psychiatric drugs starting with Thorazine swept the scene. Soon, anybody with a fountain pen and a prescription pad could be a psychiatrist; seven years of specialist training were no longer required. Hope was soon raised that psychosis would next follow the example of tuberculosis, first with effective patient treatment, and evolving later into the closing of highly expensive specialty hospitals.

Fads and Fashions. Many of these changes did result in general savings. In each step in the therapeutic process, the leadership of the specialty were thrown into disarray by radically new treatments requiring many years of re-training to master. Brash young physicians displaced the experienced older ones; the older ones never quite got it, and the younger ones never quite got over it. The ultimate outcome of this uproar was what you can now see in the center of many cities: "homeless" people living in rags on steam grates, because there are few psychiatric hospitals for chronic indigents, anymore. And basically, no good ways to define and reimburse psychiatrists.

Trust Fund Babies. The effect on upper-class "trust fund baby" patients is harder to notice, but inevitably young people of any class will outlive their parents, and often outlive the trust fund as well. What did further disrupt the vulnerable changing treatment scene, was the introduction of large numbers of addicts to recreational drugs, which tended to affect those who could afford the cost, sooner than those who could not. The system was disrupted from the top down at first, and then it became a regular feature of the youth scene for young people of any social class. The closing of upper-class inpatient facilities is particularly disruptive when the signs of addiction first make their appearance, encountering a distraught family having no familiarity with what to expect, or whatever treatment facilities are available, however abundant or scarce, good or bad.

Non-Relatedness of Psychiatric Severity to Hospitalization. There is an old saying in psychiatric circles: "People aren't hospitalized because they have psychiatric conditions. They are hospitalized because they are bothering somebody." Because psychiatry at the time was regarded as a state responsibility rather than a federal one, there were enormous disparities in treatment adequacy. It should be recognized that interstate disparities are part of the force behind the move to federalize. It's actually one of the pressures by interest groups to upgrade spending in poor states, which in time will correct the imbalances between states which James Madison envisioned as a driving force for change. Because California was particularly generous, it was punished by attracting large numbers of psychiatric patients. The response of neighboring states was quite the opposite; they closed what few state facilities survived, and the patients drifted to California. In both cases, local politicians found something to boast about, and their opponents found something to complain about.

The Rather Drastic Philadelphia Method. One place they couldn't quite boast of, was the relative absence of drug addiction in Philadelphia, for quite a long time. The local Mafia chieftain declared anyone selling drugs in his territory wouldn't even live to regret it. His methods were easy to notice, and for a number of years Philadelphia was "clean". The proof that this was the cause was easily demonstrated by an upsurge in drug addicts soon after a neighboring Mafia tribe "bumped him off".

Cycles. One psychiatric social worker looked on the scene with disgust, and offered this explanation. "These psychiatric fads come and go, and they always will. We see patients on steam grates and we say they must be hospitalized to get better treatment. After a while, we call those hospitals 'snake pits' and then say the patients should be integrated back into society." That was her view of it, and everybody else except me may be right. But I feel blame for the present mess is partly shared among many forces: To over-enthusiasm for a new treatment, partly stimulated by a desire to save a lot of public money which encourages a suspension of disbelief, and adverse

"John Kennedy closed the Snake Pits. Who will close the steam grates?"

decisions made by public officials, with other priorities being pressed upon them. Increasing longevity caused adverse de-selection to emerge from state governments funding nursing homes for the indigent elderly, for example. We unfortunately do need some bad examples to trigger improvement, but too many of them will overwhelm a government into seeing no way out except hunkering down.

The End of the Dream Economy The shift in American international trade payments from positive to negative, which took place around 1966 reminded us we weren't as rich as we thought we were, while the recreational drug scene shifted attention to different clients for psychiatric care. The two movements have a certain amount in common. In other words, the nation shifted charitable priorities away from chronic psychosis. It was a result of a whole host of pressures independent of the inclinations of the psychiatric patients and the psychiatric doctors. Psychiatry is an extreme case, because the patients always surrender a certain amount of autonomy. But it is a warning to everyone that it is dangerous to surrender the remaining control of your fate to people who have limited incentive to look out for your interests. I have been convinced by the arguments that the closing of high-class, high-cost psychiatric hospitals for the rich, did not start this trend. But when wealthy powerful people cannot find an institution they are perfectly willing to pay for, (as is now true in the case of chronic adult psychosis), it is a remarkable development. And it raises a question how much further this trend might go.

That Dratted DRG, Again. Hospital payment by diagnosis makes a reasonable assumption that hospitalization costs are somehow related to the diagnosis, but while that's often true it is seldom precise. The less the precision of the diagnosis, the less precision it will have in determining cost. When it reaches the extreme of two million diagnosis categories lumped into two hundred diagnosis-related groups, it is inevitable that some diagnoses are unrelated to the mean, in the services they require. Furthermore, some patients with identical diagnoses have complications involving fresh departures in treatment. Or they will be affected by unusual manifestations of illness requiring them to run up special costs. Variations are sometimes enough to bankrupt a family, sometimes they are so extreme they bankrupt a hospital. Bigger hospitals find the law of large numbers often takes care of the problem, but combined with local environmental or politician problems, sometimes even a very big hospital can be shaken by an epidemic.

Outliers. That is, "outliers" will be found, where the DRG payment is not even remotely appropriate. But the main reason DRG is adequate for most hospitals, is the payer wills it to be so, and the hospital then devises some work-around which the payer chooses not to notice. In the case of psychiatry, whole disciplines of illness are occasionally found to have little association between diagnosis and cost of treatment. No matter what his diagnosis may be, a person who thinks he is Napoleon can stay in a hospital for one day, or his whole life, depending on circumstances. So the DRG law at first provided outliers should be paid the old way, by itemized services, for psychiatry and other outliers. That was once the way we paid for all hospitalizations, so why wouldn't it continue to suffice for outliers to be treated as exceptions? The flaw in this reasoning, of course, was prices of individual services were discretionary, and pretty much limited to exceptional cases, plus psychiatry. That led to two clusters of prices in the chargemaster lists, one for outliers in conventional general hospitals, and a second one for psychiatric hospitals. Either way, it seemed a good precaution to set the prices high.

Strained State Budgets. In government circles, there is a standard sort of behavior, usually tolerated as a normal part of the negotiations. To get a bill passed in Congress without delay, technical adjustments can come later. In retrospect, it is unclear whether readjustments were bungled or whether the problem was unsolvable; the payers' fuse did seem to have been rather short. In any event, when the number of psychiatric beds fell toward 40,000 from an earlier 500,000, many gave up and went out of business.

Windfall, Then Disaster. And so it came about in those days that general hospitals were chafed by low prices set for DRG, while psychiatric hospitals were effectively given blank checks, and prospered notoriously. A movement was even under discussion, to move non-psychiatric patients into psychiatric hospitals, but events headed this off. It took some time for all of this to work through the system, but eventually three situations survived. Prices were drastically reduced for psychiatric DRGs, to the point where hospitals of this type were driven out of business. Secondly, the DRG system proved to be a highly efficient rationing system, eventually moving toward a pattern of 2% profit margins within a 2% national inflation rate. And thirdly, the Chargemaster rates remained high, discouraging hospitalization and encouraging outpatients. One by one, famous established psychiatric facilities closed their doors, to the point where indigent patients are found on steam grates, and some affluent ones, too.

The Veterans Administration. As a matter of fact, there is one place left to treat inpatient psychiatric patients – the Veteran's Administration hospital system, if you can find an empty bed. The bed capacity is small, but at least they do not segregate by ability to pay. Social workers desperately looking for somewhere to place psychiatric patients, quickly learned to ask the most important question first: "Have you ever been a veteran?" If so, regardless of income, but somewhat dependent on locality, it is one lucky patient. All of the inadequacies of the VA informal rationing system soon come to light, however; the long waiting lists, remoteness of location, the recreational drug epidemic, the demoralized staff. With thousands of patients on their outpatient waiting lists, it was just not possible to cover all this up, to say nothing of fixing it before newspaper reporters arrive. Newsmedia have generally been ardent supporters of Obamacare and government-run medical care, but even they have been chastened by the example of it encountered in the Veteran's Administration. Let me help them with their outrage. The Armed Forces themselves will have nothing to do with VA, running an independent system of military hospitals for active-duty military, and politicians they wish to court. When President Eisenhower had a heart attack, he went to Walter Reed Hospital, Franklin Roosevelt and a host of other presidents went to the Naval Hospital in Bethesda. Even Senator Joe McCarthy died in the Naval Hospital, where the first thing a VIP says is, "No one must know I am here." That's the motto of military hospitals. But if any important government official is ever cared for in a Veteran's Hospital, by contrast, it will be very big news, indeed.

Health Insurance Companies Reach for the Brass Ring

I n the light of future developments, we might someday look back on the University of Pittsburgh as the place health insurance stepped over a line, and merged group practices with health insurance companies. It's true that was somewhat the way the first Blue Cross in Houston, Texas, had been organized, although it eventually split into component parts. It's the thought running through closed-panel insurance that this might be an easy way to circumvent antitrust laws, because vertical integration is no longer considered a *per se* violation. Although, as mentioned earlier, it isn't necessarily a good thing either, and it isn't immune to a trial of the facts.

It has certainly aroused violent discomfort among excluded competitors in allied industries, to allow mediation control to fall into the hands of a corporation which could profit from the favoritism. Better to conduct arms-length transactions; the regulator should not profit from its own decisions. No law exactly says this should be so; the customers just like it better. And indeed Pittsburgh was the location of the defining court case, decades ago, where non-profit organizations were declared exempt from antitrust suits, just as Philadelphia had the first case which declared an end to charitable immunity. Until someone re-litigates these cases in a changed environment, these old court decisions retain a particularly large impact on local thinking.

Red tape is always expensive, and right now high costs are a challenging problem. Furthermore, big business is currently paying the bill, and big business would like to be satisfied on the point. That raises another historical point. Henry Kaiser gets credit for inventing the employer-based tax exemption, but the issue was rampant in all of the steel industry, which was often the leader in such innovations. The steel industry has pretty well abandoned America and gone to the Far East except for steel made out of scrap. The health insurance companies traditionally jumped at the command of the big employers, but maybe there is an opportunity for a revision of leadership in the industrial unions, particularly in steel. But while it may well be true this political vacuum has been filled with new leadership, it is likely some old traditions persist. The bitterness of the Molly Maguire era was thought to have ended a century ago,

> *"Red tape is always expensive."*

but if your ancestor was hanged or assassinated, the legend lives on. Sounds sort of like the Balkans, doesn't it? Some people in Bosnia are still endorsing genocide in retaliation for Thirteenth century church burnings.

Based on reasonings of this sort, it is fair to conclude that even if big business (or big government) changes its mind about the ultimate outcome, this kind of behavior may or may not change. Uncertain of the eventual outcome, both providers and vendors of care may think it is better to leave the matter alone. And if someone else pays the bill, someone else may decide to change the system of utilization control. Through a convoluted history in several steps, the University of Pittsburgh has formed a large salaried group practice, and merged it with the captive teaching hospital at one end, and the captive health insurance company at the other. Pennsylvania is a large state with rather wide sociological and industrial differences, but it is only natural that the other medical schools, hospitals, physician groups and insurance companies would worry that this system might migrate into their neighboring territories. At the very least, rearrangements on such a large scale would be expensive and complicated. And not necessarily beneficial to the common good.

In case the reasoning isn't clear, let us restate the argument which was persuasive to the United States Supreme Court in the case of *State Oil v. Kahn*. As conglomerates acquire new businesses, they find they are not particularly good at managing a few parts of the whole. It is failure in those defective components, which brings the whole conglomerate enterprise, down.

Companies may merge across traditional occupational boundaries, for a variety of reasons. One of the most questionable reasons to merge, is to eliminate an unwelcome constraint on your plans, such as a new invention. Another would be to eliminate a critic whose views thwart you for reasons you do not understand. In the present situation, a medical school which supplies new physicians to a region should not be allowed to favor or control its graduates, or to enhance, protect or destroy their environment, particularly if the public suffers from the effects of it. When a medical conglomerate is allowed to profit in some of its divisions, in spite of losing money in others, the interests of the conglomerate may not be parallel with the interests of the public, in their choices of winners and losers. A mixture of taxable and nontaxable activities offer many opportunities for this to be the result.

Academia Gets Its Share of Blame

In 910, Abraham Flexner produced a book-long report on reforming medical education, under the sponsorship of the American Medical Association and the funding of the Carnegie Institution. The report was a product of the progressive era of reform which ended the Gilded Age, and can fairly be described as the handbook of a revolution in American medicine. The book had the impact on closing 106 of the 160 medical schools in the United States and Canada. To Flexner that was a disappointment; he thought only 31 were worth saving. To be a good doctor, in his opinion, required between six and eight years of scientific training. The quality of student as well as the quality of schools was important, justifying a vast shrinkage of the student body. He liked research and unleashed an avalanche of medical research which subsequently transformed medical care in a hundred ways.

Having said all that, it must be acknowledged, Abe Flexner had been educated in Germany, and his efforts mainly crystallized the transfer of German academic medicine to America, and from here onward to the world. What's being acknowledged is that for a time, German Medicine was far ahead of us, in an environment where we aspired to be the leaders.

"Abner Flexner, the Rainmaker."
German Model for Medical Schools

Flexner was a charismatic figure, supported by American Medical Association reports from its Council of Medical Education, the wealth of the Carnegie Institution, and the enormous resources of the Rockefeller

Foundation. American academic medicine pointed to the example of the Johns Hopkins Medical School, formed before the ferment of pre-World War I, and now being given prominence by Teddy Roosevelt, Woodrow Wilson and the rest of the muckraking era who aspired to replace the Gilded Age with something better. America was aching to take charge of something, had great gobs of philanthropic money at its disposal, and the wind in its sails. Abraham Flexner was a towering figure, all right, but he was not a physician, an academic, or a scientist. He was more the agent of revolution than its originator, ending up as the patron saint of several political factions, individually fighting academic wars with each other. He was, in short, a rain-maker.

Abe Flexner and his book aimed to reduce the number of medical schools from 160 to 31, demanding the survivors look like German schools. This was not so strange; like Japan and China today competing with America, Flexner wanted to compete with Germany more than he wanted to worship it. The students of his dreams were required to be college graduates, the curriculum was to be four years long with two years of science followed by two years of hands-on learning. If the school could afford it, the professors would be on full-time salary, freed of any need to practice in order to make a living. On this last point, many beg to differ, arguing you have to get on a boat to learn how to sail one. There were many echoes of the ferment to come, in the upheavals of the 1960's, and Humboldt's University of Berlin was the source of quite a few, in both cases.

Immediately there arose a town-and-gown competition. The gown group had the point they could afford the time to do some research. The town group had the point you couldn't teach doctors if you weren't one, yourself. The distinction is probably best understood by comparing medical students with law students. Both were originally taught by practitioners; schools were late arrivals. Many lawyers have remarked that a law school graduate now knows almost nothing about the practice of law until he joins a firm which teaches it to him. A medical student (post-Flexner) can do a pretty good job with most medical problems, the day he graduates. The practicing physicians have retreated into specialty training; a doctor has trouble becoming a specialist if he didn't have the right residency. The rest of the awe-inspiring march of medical progress in the Twentieth century, is the consequence of pouring unbelievable amounts of money into the system, thereby attracting a glittering array of talented medical students. Some of the talent is unbelievable. My own medical school, as an example, has a symphony orchestra made up of students in their spare time, performing on a truly professional level for their own amusement. In a sense, all of this was due to Flexner. In another sense, Flexner himself had little to do with originating it.

Now, forget the yellow journalism, or muckraking, quality of what I am about to relate. A book was recently published relating that a particular medical school was able to support its operations without touching a penny of medical student tuition for ten consecutive years. Instead, the tuition money was transferred to the University's undergraduate schools, and the medical school subsisted on research and other funds. The undergraduates continue to protest about rich doctors, while the medical students complain about going a hundred thousand into debt – to pay their tuition. But forget that part. The most undesirable situation it reflects is that for ten years, the school was totally able to exclude any parent and student influence in an area that unfortunately has a growing power over events, the school's finances. If the students, families and alumni of a university have no power to influence its decisions, who does have such power?

Sometimes, Even the Supreme Court Looks Negligent

If the United States Supreme Court makes a mistake, it remains pretty much a mistake in residence until the Court itself re-examines the matter. It would be indelicate for anyone else to cite a list of examples for this observation, so they are customarily taken up one at a time, at considerable expense. The desirable re-examination with the greatest consequence to Healthcare would be the 1982 decision in *State of Arizona v. Maricopa County Medical Society.*

Maricopa County is where Phoenix is located in Arizona, and its County Medical Society was one of the pioneers in what were then called Foundations for Medical Care. These were organizations in which local physicians took the lead in organizing and managing health insurance for the local community. The rules and policies of the Foundations were conceived and implemented by physicians, who were dismayed by the consequences of defects in health financing they could see in daily practice. Except for this physician dominance, it would be fair to say that Foundations for Medical Care were about the same as what we now call HMOs. It is also true these physicians were impatient with both the government and the health insurance companies, who seemed to resist helping the sick poor by implying it might violate some *per se* technicality aimed at business corporations. As the lame excuse would have it, our hands are tied. The obvious fact is someone in Arizona didn't like physicians, or didn't like what they were threatening to do.

An agreement among competitors to lower prices for the poor, is after all not exactly the same anti-competitive behavior, as a "contrivance" to raise prices for your own benefit. It seemed most unfortunate to lump it together with its opposite as "per se" violations, requiring no examination of the evidence to distinguish the two. And furthermore, on the topic of regulating business corporations, it is not exactly an enumerated Constitutional power of the federal government, to amend the Constitution by treating all corporations as essentially identical, or lowering prices the same as raising them. The whole anti-Foundation movement sounds pretty spurious.

At the same time, "Foundation" physicians believed they could see opportunities for reducing waste in the local hospitals which would only be exploited if physicians were in charge, because physicians could sense the cost/benefit more readily than anyone else. Having recently returned from the Korean War, these doctors knew medical care could be excellent even without such a thing as health insurance, and indeed even if hospitals were only a collection of tents. Perhaps a few of them were overly influenced by the TV serial, "MASH", whose central theme is that if doctors take the lead and do the right thing, much can be forgiven. That's a sort of Hollywood restatement of the latitude of ancient Courts of Equity, charged with finding a way to achieve Justice – to cover a situation where obvious harm exists, but no law exactly addresses it.

97

Accordingly, the "better sort" of doctor in Arizona believed they perceived the respectable doctors would readily agree to care for the poor at lower rates, whereas the shirkers in their midst would ruin things for everybody by refusing to do a fair share of *pro bono* work. Like labor unions, the doctors greatly resented the free rider phenomenon.

The idea of a two-class system of medical care was also abhorrent to them, however; if there wasn't enough money to spread around, a "good" doctor would just agree to lower his fees unilaterally. This moral quarrel often conflicts American business, which takes the view that it doesn't really matter what costs or taxes or burdens are imposed by government. What matters to big business is that all competitors need to abide by the same handicaps. When handicaps are roughly equal, the difference between success and failure is – talent. But the contrast between that and the antitrust position of individual tradesmen has never been satisfactorily defined.

To a considerable degree, talent rising to the top summarizes the aspirations of the anti-trust statutes, where it regularly becomes a source of both suppression and escalation of prices. Physicians are ultimately expected, not least by their colleagues, to find their highest duty is fiducial to the patients' best interest, particularly when the main conflict is merely a financial one. A corporation, by contrast, has a primary duty to its shareholders, who can sue them if they put benevolence ahead of profit. A corporation is a contract between the State and the shareholders, quite the reverse of the duty of government to its individual citizens. In the anti-trust arena, the contrast between citizen and corporation is jumbled. Particularly in the case of the *per se* violations, the difference between a business corporation and a medical society is quite wide enough to justify considerable professional latitude. As it is not, in the case of insurers, and as it only partly remains, in the case of hospitals. Anti-trust statutes could have a real value in distinguishing borders between individual tradesmen and various groupings of them, but so far the distinctions are far from reasonable. The Maricopa Medical Society responded with perhaps excessive enthusiasm to the challenge of making local sense out of a price-fixing dilemma, but it was never given the opportunity to make its case.

At one time, local healthcare costs were suppressed by imposing competition on the hospitals, holding insurance administrators to be mindless clerks to pay the bills, not as cup-bearers of fairness in a naughty world. Needless to say, the hospitals and health insurers had long chafed at the ability of physicians to switch hospitals freely, and the patients to switch insurers, whereas Arizona's Attorney General seemed to suspect some vague return to Robin Hood notions of a special right to defy the law. Somehow the ancient concept of professional latitude has been supplanted as inconvenient to the goals of competitors. In certain parts of the country, big business is already expanding its financial control of hospitals and insurers, into acting as agents for assuring high quality medical care, while suppressing its cost. On Wall Street, such behavior is quickly seen and labeled as "talking up your book of business". With the defeat of physicians by the Maricopa decision, plus the withdrawal of big business owners from identifiable management roles, the way was soon opened for hospitals and insurance companies to assert unrestrained control of their own finances. Thirty years later, hospitals and insurers are now universally merging, and applying selective controls over admitting pliant physicians as their employees. The Affordable Care Act is the mechanism by which government interjects a new layer of control, thereby converting government itself into the new hidden battlefield. It seems a very far cry from leaving medical decisions in the hands of physicians and their patients, to choose treatments, and to agree on their price.

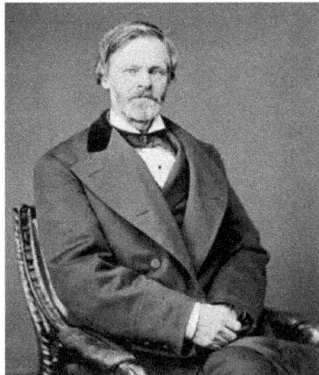

Sen. John Sherman

The Attorney General of Arizona, himself a colorful character, soon brought suit for anti-trust violation, since price-fixing was a declared *per se* violation, or identification of the absence of competition. These were additions made to the Sherman Anti-Trust Act by earlier Supreme Courts, who found an Act first written on the back of an envelope was lacking in regulations. Further strictures were imposed by the Clayton Anti-Trust Act, but these both might be remedied by subsequent Congresses, and thus lacked appropriate majesty. The crucial consequence was that the District Court of Arizona found it quite unnecessary to hold a trial or hear the evidence. The Court found against the doctors entirely on the basis of a motion for summary judgment. The matter then passed through the Court of Appeals to the Supreme Court, which on the theory that price fixing is price fixing, on a vote of 4 to 3, upheld the Arizona suit. All the way from a writ of summary judgment in a district court, to the United States Supreme Court, without formal examination of the facts. If either of the two absent members eligible to vote, had voted, it is certainly mathematically possible for the decision to have gone the other way.

Perhaps, strictly on lawyerisms, that was safely correct. But in terms of the effect on medical care, it won the war for control of hospitals and the insurance companies which began with Abraham Flexner's beatification of college-educated physicians. Somehow *Maricopa* was interpreted to mean that a hospital or an insurance company might do many medical things which were forbidden to organizations run by physicians. The consequence is Foundations run by physicians are under constant threat of what might happen to them if they do what HMOs are now seen to be doing every day. The whole Clinton health fracas revolved around this particular case and its implications. From the physician point of view, if you had medical training, you had been disqualified from running a Health Maintenance Organization, because a change of leadership seems to shift the antitrust issue to a different level within two identical organizations. And that was true even if the physician had been trained for the role, while the administrator had not.

What was particularly galling was to be tarred with the brush of antitrust, whereas others could describe identical behavior as self-disciplined and in the public interest. Self-imposed financial restraint was taunted and abused by aspirants for the same job with the same temptations, with multi-million dollar incomes, but without adherence to the same code of ethics. The emerging joke is that after the Clinton Healthcare Plan's uproar, the public decided they disliked HMO's intensely, mainly because they couldn't choose their own doctor, and the doctor was being hampered in doing what seemed professionally best for the patient. None of these legal issues had significantly arisen for physician-run HMOs. While of course that outcome might appear, such disputes would be settled by physicians, using medical arguments, followed by a change in management if the medical community at large, widely disagreed with the decision. The only substantial difference was that doctors were running one organization but subservient in the other, and the Courts had found that whenever doctors were in charge it amounted to price-fixing between competitors. As matters eventually turned out, the hospitals resolved this battle by converting nearly all practicing physicians into their employees, and the war has now shifted to who will control hospitals.

It now remains for some case to be found and carried to the Supreme Court which might allow an examination of the facts of this matter, perhaps remanding the case back to the District Court to hold a trial. That would seem a bare minimum after thirty years, even though now it might no longer address precisely the same issue. Somehow, a way must be found to examine which of two rather extreme theories of the Wild Wild West needs to be laughed off. Either we must re-examine whether, always and everywhere, price-fixing is such an undiluted evil it never requires an examination of the evidence. Or whether the absence of identifiable harm introduces a balancing need to question such judgments, when made under professional circumstances.

While on the subject of mixing business practices with professional standards, we might as well direct judicial attention to the unfair and probably (equal justice) unconstitutional tax preference for employers who purchase health insurance for their employees, to enjoy a huge corporate tax saving themselves by doing so. Not merely for the benefit of the employees, which is much discussed, but a usually much greater financial benefit for the shareholders when the corporate tax level is high enough. An unnecessary grievance is created for millions of self-employed and unemployed people who lack this tax shelter, and also for the owners of usually much smaller business enterprises, who must compete with them.

It might be argued that double taxation of corporations inevitably provides the loophole of double tax-exemption, and even this would often understate the discrepancy because of the differences in marginal rates. Lack of participation in this double tax benefit, is arguably a main obstacle to extending employee health insurance to others, or even substituting a superior health payment methodology. Now seventy years old, this grievance can be regarded, not only as having dubious evasions at its historical origin, but has resisted multiple efforts for repeal, and distorts the relative lifestyles of the two main participants in the workforce: small, and large, businesses. Henry Kaiser claimed he once had difficulty attracting employees to his West Coast war industries because of wartime wage and price controls, an excuse which should have ended the practice in 1945. Lack of a review-and-reconstruction of this bizarre lobbying product could potentially distort the application of the Affordable Care Act, in ways which are impossible to foresee. Indefinite enshrinement of the legal principles in this tangle, particularly the indefinite postponement of its resolution, could reverberate for more decades. The fringe-benefits circumvention for example has since grown entirely out of control, while it is fiercely defended by business and union interests. As it grows, however, the inequity to the self-employed and unemployed by remaining excluded from it, also grows.

Summary of the Maricopa Case

From a legal standpoint, the most uncomfortable feature of the case of the Maricopa Medical Society is that it went all the way to the Supreme Court without any trial of the facts or real opportunity for the defendants to present their case. That is, the whole HMO movement was effectively removed from the hands of physicians by a motion for summary judgment, on a Supreme Court decision, 4 to 3. It would be interesting to learn the attitudes of the remaining two Justices who recused themselves, but who could have reversed it.

To hold a trial of the facts by remanding the case for trial, would seem to be one easy way to introduce the defense which the doctors would have made. It could be improper to suggest to their lawyers what the defense should now be, because new officers of the Medical Society might hold different opinions. The Medicaid Act was passed in 1965, requiring state consent for a jointly administered program. By 1972, Arizona was the only remaining state not to have agreed to Medicaid, which by then was widely recognized as the worst run and most underfunded medical program in America. In 1982, Arizona adopted a small portion of Medicaid, and it was only in 1988 that it fully adopted the program. In 2001, Arizona's governor was offered 7.9 billion dollars over four years, as matching money for the insurance exchange feature of the Affordable Care Act, which by then heavily absorbed the Medicaid program. The Governor recommended to the Legislature that they accept the offer, because at least it was "better than Medicaid". There can be little doubt the Legislature of Arizona was adamant on the issue. And the Medicaid program is certainly better funded than it formerly was. But the central feature of Medicaid's HMO remains that of the Maricopa decision: its policies and administration are not directed by physicians. On the issue of whether control should rest with payers or professionals, payers prevailed.

What were the doctors expected to do with sick poor people? No doubt, there was a wide divergence of opinion, but it must have seemed likely to someone, only a handful of saintly volunteers would now step forward, and none of them would be willing to pay hospitals their list prices. There is some truth to the last part. The doctors felt it would only work by shaming a substantial majority of their own members into accepting the cases at discount prices, and the only weapon they had was to make it a condition for membership in the medical society. That might once have been a powerful incentive, but systematic undermining of its powers has now made it more questionable whether it could still succeed in its original plan. At the time of the first trial, there was probably enough slack in hospital revenue to cover the indigent need. With a changed economy, the premise needs to be tested more hesitantly.

Under these contentious circumstances surely the Supreme Court could, even now, find some words to devise a better outcome. Price fixing is a *per se* violation of the act, and there is little doubt that all HMOs now fix prices. Only a physician-run HMO can be accused of "fixing" prices too low for competitive reasons, although it has always been arguable how strongly they would naturally compete for indigent patients. The Supreme Court may be reluctant to overrule the price fixing part because of the spill-over effect of a century of custom, and the Arizona politics of this case are surely thorny.

As time passes, the *Maricopa* case is fast becoming as dignified by long standing, as the price "fixing" notions were when it all started. Surely, at least the Court could find some clarifying language about physician-run HMOs as *obiter dicta*. The response of the non-physician-run HMOs was to exploit the opportunity to eliminate the competition of physician-run groups within the price-fixed arena. In the meantime, however, the public has found HMOs run by non-physicians have become contentious in the extreme, whereas the earlier physician-run Foundations for Medical Care were tolerated by most physicians, and embraced by quite a few. The matter is one of the important threads in the Obamacare controversy, so the Supreme Court has an opportunity to improve quite a few situations by writing a clarifying paragraph or two.

The Coming End to Ink Blots.

Medicare spends about $56 billion a year. The National Institutes of Health spends $30 billion, rising at a rate of 3% a year, or about the national inflation rate. Full disclosure: I was an employee of the NIH for two years, and think highly of the place. The Director of NIH at that time was James Shannon, who had been in charge of the New York division of Goldwater Hospital on Welfare Island in New York harbor, while I was a medical student on the Columbia division of the same hospital. I didn't meet Shannon in New York, but I heard everyone who knew him, speak with awe. The big news when I was a student was that he had accepted a job in the commercial drug industry, which was deemed a degrading sell-out. There was much cluck-clucking, which medical students intended as giving the drug industry a not-so-subtle warning from us their betters, that we would never, ever, consider such a sell-out to the moneychangers. Shannon persisted in the drug industry for a few years, and then turned up as Director of the NIH.

He never confided his goals to me, but it was widely reported he only accepted the political job, on condition Congress would absolutely never introduce political goals into the research process. No scientist would ever be forced to study a project because some Congressman's wife had a disease, or thought she did. Grants would absolutely never be awarded with a geopolitical bias, and the consideration of favoring a particular drug company's research leads, would absolutely never be tolerated. And indeed, the NIH was pretty much run on such starchy principles for at least fifteen years. By the end of that period, its reputation was immense.

During that period, the grounds of the NIH in Bethesda grew from an expansive, golf course-like, estate with only a billion or so budget, into an extensive little city of research buildings, with traffic lights and uniformed policemen to direct traffic. And, a $30 billion budget whose composition is not easy to come by, but only 10% of which is reported to be spent in-house. The greatest proportion of the budget is now dispensed to far-flung academia in the form of grants. The emphasis of current research can be inferred from its list of specified targets, which concentrate on cancer, antibiotic resistance, brain disorders and Alzheimer's disease. A few years ago, HIV/AIDS was targeted, and so successfully, it dropped off the targeted list. Let me tell you a trade secret about research: most proposed research is a waste of money, accomplishing little. The art of selecting which proposal to fund is therefore a difficult one, but there is no doubt some scientists are better at both selecting it and doing it than others; only about 20% of grant requests are selected to be funded. How many potential Nobel prizes are in the rejected 80% is unknown, but there must be some.

"What will follow protein chemistry?"

Successful researchers quite often prove to be high-stakes gamblers, and some people seem to have better hunches than others. Some people just don't have the right temperament, but it's pretty hard to identify just what that is. On the other hand, some people only flourish when surrounded by others with the "right stuff", while others work best when left alone in solitude. I hate to say it, but a few people also excel at the fine art of stealing the ideas of others with less drive and energy. Some people burn out at an early age, others keep producing good work past the retirement age. All in all, it's probably remarkable that the 20% who are selected, produce so much. But since so much time and money comes to nothing, the environment is a dangerous one, rather glibly leading to a conversational conclusion that someone else should have got the grant. On the other hand, we have made it possible to become a billionaire before you are thirty, so some real pirates get attracted to research. Observations of this general sort lead me to believe, if we should suddenly get the announcement of a cheap effective cure for cancer, there would immediately be a chorus of voices, demanding next year's NIH budget be cut in half. And the frustrating thing would be, no one could be entirely sure that was wrong.

That summarizes one way this promenade could end; not with a whimper, but a bang. A famous success, with prizes and speeches and even statues – followed by a steep budget cut. The other way, would be the slow exhaustion of contemporary protein chemistry, followed by nothing which could match it for glamor. For the past twenty years, the five hundred peer-selected papers chosen for presentation at prestigious three-day research seminars – have overwhelmingly shown slides displaying ink blots.

Let me explain. Until twenty years ago, most successful new drugs and biochemical discoveries have involved small molecules. It seemed clear most of the remaining secrets were hidden in the coils and recesses of protein chemistry, but protein chemistry was just too hard to do quickly. We spent a billion dollars exploring the human genome, only to find it explained no more than 2% of disease. So we doubted the research and repeated it, spending another billion to no avail. Almost all these experiments involved chromatography, so almost all of the experiments showed their results as blots on a piece of paper, rather uniformly resembling ink blots in a psychiatric personality test. Either a novel bulge appeared, or two sets of bulges (amazingly) showed no difference in bulges. After twenty years of watching slides showing ink blots, I retired from the scene and started clinical practice and writing books.

When a new miracle is discovered, its particular ink blot will probably look a lot like other ink blots, so why go to so many meetings. It looks to me as though ink blots of mitochondria, or ink blots of Golgi bodies will demonstrate the new miracle, or else every conceivable ink blot will be performed on those particles, and nothing striking will turn up. Somewhere, some cure for cancer and Alzheimer's disease will exist, but its effect need not be demonstrated in its protein chromatography. But at least until the cure is found, or every imaginable ink blot has been photographed, the ink blot parade will continue, and then it will gradually wear out. At least to me, it seems incredible the present approach can continue much longer. What I'm saying is we need a new cure fast, or else we need a new experimental tool.

There's another danger I haven't mentioned. Like the cost overruns of clinical practice, the best place to direct the accountants who count the beans of research grants, is the indirect overhead. It's characteristic for grants to come as direct and indirect costs, and the indirect costs are approximately 70% of the direct ones. Research institutes who operate on a for-profit basis all agree that 70% is if anything far too little, and the non-profits nod in agreement. It sure doesn't feel appropriate to give the administration of academia a 70% cushion for the library, air conditioning, etc, necessary to sustain these billions of dollars for research. Sooner or later, someone will apply the old government technique for dealing with an expense account you don't understand: Cut its indirect overhead budget 10% and see what happens. If nothing bad seems to happen, cut it 10% more. And so forth until you have starved it to death, forced it to commit suicide, or identified its legitimacy. No, don't do it. Either you do research or you don't, and if you want the right answer you must do it the right way. But if Shannon's rules are egregiously flouted, disaster will more likely be the consequence.

After the Second World War, America decided to do what only America could afford to do. We decided to spend astonishing amounts of money, curing disease. The unproven theory for gambling this enormous fortune was – in the long run, it would cost less than subsidizing everybody to be treated in old-fashioned ways. And it really has been shown to work. In 1950 we had 500,000 state and municipal hospital beds for mental disorder. Today, we only have about 40,000. Can you imagine how much money that has saved? Or the 100,000 beds for tuberculosis? Or the fifty thousand beds for polio? What is left to do is treat about five diseases of late-life onset, and there is a reasonable chance to do it in the next two decades. Just double those numbers, and you still have a bargain. Yes, it's true we have not resorted to expedients every other civilized nation in the world has resorted to, and yes it is true the medical profession will never be the same. But this is America, right? We plan to give it away to all those other civilized nations, mostly free, to foreigners who might never dream of doing the same for us. That's part of the overachieving American character, too.

Psychiatry: Scientific Frontier, or Stormy Seas?

Although scientific news about healthcare research is mostly pretty good, a storm may be approaching in psychiatry. Not only are that specialty's finances in disarray, but as the rest of the profession steadily conquers its share of diseases, lack of progress in psychiatry becomes more noticeable. Large sums are donated and granted to repair this gap, in a typically American approach to such obstacles. Maybe it is too soon to expect dramatic results. President John Kennedy once learned thorazine was helping psychotic people go home from state mental hospitals, and put that information alongside the painful cost of maintaining 500,000 rather decrepit beds. Effectively, he closed most of them. It was well intentioned, but too quick. The important thing to notice was how very many psychotic patients there were, and therefore how big a job it entails.

Responding to investigative reporters who interviewed the inner city "skid rows" and wrote magazine articles about them, most of them were razed, gentrified, and those patients who were unsuitable for living independently, were dispersed into other community living. I had a number of them in the accident room as patients, and it was my observation that most were not alcoholics at all, but mentally deranged. An army of young hopefuls were recruited into a new profession of mental rehabilitation, and were viewed with suspicion by contemporaries who went into more traditional specialties. In time, the polarization between these two groups became a noticeable feature of political life. It began to be evident that political machines had always attracted some mentally unstable hangers-on, and the candidates themselves tended toward egotism of a degree not always useful. Nothing new, here, but it somehow heated up as politics lost attraction as an entertainment, compared with new competitors.

Around 1965, the recreational drug scene along with its flower children and colorful activists unexpectedly hit us, trailed by optimistic news reports that heroin really wasn't so bad, LSD might have therapeutic potentials, and marijuana might even be beneficial compared with alcohol. Some of these contentions have been scientifically dismissed, but one discovery was greeted with delight by school children: marijuana was about the same as alcohol, but the smell on the breath didn't give it away. For a while, it was unclear whether drugs made you psychotic, or psychotic people were attracted to drugs; it's still not entirely clear.

The city police, who were dragooned into maintaining law and order amidst this commotion, resorted to the only resource they had, which was the local jails. The public agreed, perhaps hoping to scare the miscreant children, and passed laws about speedy trials for drug offenders, mandatory jail sentencing, and mandatory long sentences. The prisons filled up, older prisoners taught newcomers some tricks, and it was not long before the prison systems and the school systems were destabilized. We closed the snake pits and skid rows, all right, but we gave ourselves a drug problem, a prison problem, and a school problem.

The simultaneous development of a problem we had never quite seen before, at least to anything like a similar degree, caused a few reflective people to remember we had always had a large segment who were mentally unstable. It was a tenth of the population, possibly even a fifth. My pristine suburb spends 8% of its budget on "Special" education. Some of this was indeed new. Alzheimer's disease is one of the outgrowths of the advancing longevity we are so proud of. Women who delay having children are especially prone to deliver babies with Down's syndrome of mental retardation. Women are now going to work instead of tending children and aging parents, forcing these patients more into the open. The mechanization of warfare means more rejections for mental inferiority, because soldiers need to be smart to be trusted with such weapons. So it's hard to know whether there is more mental disorder than before, or whether it has always been there, and is emerging from the shadows. In any event, we must newly face a very large segment of the population who are unemployable, and as they age, are adrift even from the discipline of regular employment.

The medical profession, preoccupied with its more usual tasks, woke up to this situation in odd little ways. One strange alert we might have noticed was the woeful inability of any medical coding system to define a relationship between psychiatric diagnosis and its treatment. In almost every other sort of condition, the diagnosis alone conveyed a pretty good idea of what the disease would cost; not in psychiatry. That was true within SNOmed and ICDA, the two main diagnostic codes for all fields of medical diagnosis, as futile efforts to squeeze it into DRG were to prove. It is also just as true within DMS (Diagnostic and Statistical Manual of Mental Disorders), the codes the psychiatric profession struggled to devise as a codebook of legitimate psychiatric conditions. It's definitely possible to construct an organized list of psychiatric diagnoses, using numerical codes instead of words. But it defies the imagination of everyone who tries it, to establish any reproducible connection between psychiatric diagnosis codes and the duration, cost or efficacy of treatments. Especially efficacy of treatments, without which little progress can be expected.

In the future, expect to hear less and less about surgery and medicine. Lots of people get sick, but sick with fewer different diseases. Research currently only seems to need to devise four or five cheap effective cures. But with psychiatry, the research is powerfully inhibited by the thick impenetrable skull, the lack of resemblance between the brain's anatomy and its functions, the extreme dangerousness of surgical experimentation, and the lack of any good idea how to connect the brain with the mind. We have a long, and expensive, way to go.

The American Health Plan; Only in America is it Imaginable

Nobody told us to do it, but let no one suppose our scientific community was the only group who had the notion. Exceptionalism likely originates deep in our culture of conquering the wild frontier. There's also the Abe Flexner or Teddy Roosevelt progressivism theory, but sometime during the winning of World War II, we Americans strongly exaggerated the idea we could do anything, and carried that idea to surprising levels. Somewhere in the course of building the atom bomb, landing a man on the moon, defeating the whole world at war, defeating the Great Depression, and winning a whole lot of Nobel Prizes, we gave ourselves the idea we really could conquer all of disease. All it seemed to require was to spend tons of money, and to set our minds not to quit. It probably is well to remember that at the time of the Bretton Woods Conference in 1944, we had two thirds of the gold in the world, locked up in Fort Knox. Foreign trade was paralyzed, because nobody else had any money.

Since 1900, average longevity has expanded from 47 years to 83. At least thirty major diseases have disappeared, fifty percent of drugs now in use were unknown just seven years ago, and so on. In 1950 we had 500,000 licensed beds for mental disorder, in 2010 only 40,000, although John Kennedy's impulsiveness probably overdid it a bit. Far from all those mental patients were transferred to jail, and far from all those jail inmates came from mental hospitals. There has been a remarkable acceleration of scientific discoveries, new drugs, new cures. And it would take more than money to do it. Why worry now about what medical care costs, when it is obvious if we cured all the diseases, even the poorest among us could easily afford to spend – nothing at all on health care. Foreigners scoff at such childish belief, but then, they retire in

> "If we cured all the diseases, even the poorest could afford to spend nothing at all on health care."

their thirties and wonder why they don't accomplish anything. Nobody ever won a war without taking casualties. You aren't listening to Quakers, when you hear that last one; the feeling isn't universal, nor is it always valid.

It does sound a little childish to go on like this, but there are signs it might actually be more or less the right path to take. We spent a billion dollars searching for cures in the genes of the entire human genome, and found very little. So we questioned the research and repeated it, spending another billion dollars. The result was unfortunately the same; apparently, that was the wrong place to look. But a man who lives in Philadelphia found thirty-seven more genes outside the cell nucleus, in the mitochondria, and spent his career finding out what they did. That sounds like a better way to go. There are scientific reasons to hope that among other things, these genes are responsible for the major diseases which make their first appearance during middle age. Four or five diseases of this sort, like cancer, diabetes, or Alzheimer's Disease, account for most of the medical costs we spend so much time worrying about. Obviously, no one is going to live forever, so there will continue to be substantial medical costs. At the very least, if we had no diseases, we would have the problem of outliving our income. Onward! Only a couple more decades to spend money, and then there will be plenty left over.

To make it last, maybe someone has to cut costs. The hospitals are the single largest source of medical spending, so somebody's unspoken plan is to let them put on fat for the coming winter, and then suddenly cut them off at the knees. After all, hotels seem to be considerably cheaper, and retirement communities run infirmaries at a fraction of the cost. We instinctively know state licensing agencies are somehow protecting some monopolies, which will disappear if we pass a few laws, although the *Maricopa* decision shows the weakness in acting on that hunch. All in favor, signify by saying aye, and it's as good as done. As somebody once said, nobody ever won a war without taking casualties.

It has been noticed by others we tend to make systematic prediction errors. If you predict what you will accomplish in a year, I'm sorry to say you can't get that much done in a year. But if you predict what will occur in twenty years, you always underestimate the enormous changes to take place in two decades. If you experiment between short-term extrapolation failures for what can change in a year, on the one hand, and imagination failures for what will take place in twenty, at the other extreme, it appears that predictions for about six years come out closest to what does actually happen. I think I got that from *The Economist.*

Will medical costs be substantially lower in six years? Probably not, but they will probably be somewhat lower, just from extending the scientific advances we have already made, to more or less everybody within our borders. Beyond that, much will depend on the scientists. Whether major discoveries will emerge, or how often, is beyond present prediction. But in five or six jumps, we can expect present accommodations to health costs, to become quite obsolete. Read the proposals to deal with them, which appear in a later section, in that light.

Although the language of exceptionalism really isn't my native language, right now the general sense it conveys, seems roughly correct. Although I'm not as reckless as some would be with research funding, I do believe the general sense of it is correct. With a little bit of luck, and considerable help from newly developed centers of foreign research, present trends do seem to be leading to a drop in both research costs and health delivery costs reasonably soon, let's say during the next generation. Improved transportation, tele-medicine and extended longevity seem to hold the promise of slimming most medical costs as we now know them. And it does seem to me reasonable to make most general hospitals into tertiary care centers, and then to shift the center of bread and butter medical care to the suburban and exurban retirement centers. Mostly, we need better transportation arrangements, to do so fairly soon.

What seems to be retaining the center of gravity in the present urban Medical Centers, seems to be: the location of research already present in those places, and the use of indigent populations for teaching purposes. When research (read: government funding) begins to dry up, it is my prediction the center of healthcare delivery will shift with the population centers, adjusted for their sickness content. My guidepost is the Hershey Medical Center, located on the most fertile farmland in the world, and only a few miles from where my ancestors lived for two hundred years. Each year I make a trip there, and every year there are more mini-mansions. A dear friend of mine advised Milton Hershey on how to build a medical school in the boonies, and frankly, all it takes is money. When present funding dries up, the center of Medicine will move to where the sickness is, unless government gets in the road of it. As far as I can predict things, it seems to mean medical care will move to retirement centers (CCRC). Some people prefer high-rise apartment buildings, but building vertically is invariably more expensive than building horizontally. Very likely, the migration of both healthcare and retirement will be dominated by making financial resources stretch further. Research? Well, research is a young person's game, so let them plan to retire earlier and become administrators later.

My ability to predict politics is poor, so I notice politicians can sometimes direct funding into wasteful directions. We might annex Canada, Mexico, and Cuba, and thereby jumble up the American economy in unrecognizable, unpredictable ways. Or we might annex Canada, Iceland, Ireland and England, for a different unpredictable future. Any of that would just be our Exceptionalism, carried out in another direction. But somebody else's exceptionalism might turn us all into a lump of molten ash, so this is a better choice. Using the same unconstrained reasoning, our leaders may decide the direction started by the careless *Maricopa* decision was ill-advised, and the people trained by the system Abraham Flexner set into motion are better qualified to run research systems, than the people elected on the second Tuesday in November. Governing this, however, will be the nature of the reaction when the taxpayers discover a few awkward things, like who benefits most when an employer gives health insurance to his employees as a tax-deductible gift.

SECTION THREE

Classical Health Saving Accounts:

Many Surprises

HEALTH SAVING ACCOUNTS

Many Surprises

One of the originators of Health Savings Accounts describes their advantages over existing health insurance. Improvements are suggested for the regular HSA. More dramatic cost improvement emerges from a lifetime HSA version, substituting whole-life approaches for pay-as-you-go. Most of this requires legislation, but could reduce health costs dramatically.

The section describes some of the nuts and bolts of Health Savings Accounts, and sketches in some more elaborate variations which might be possible. Recall we have estimated the Health Savings Accounts would earn an average 6.5% compound interest income during the long lifecycle between healthy youth and sickly elderly. But the variability of prices and terms among Catastrophic Health policies currently limits specific examples of what might be possible. And the instability of regulations explains most of the remaining uncertainties.

Classical Health Savings Accounts (C-HSA)

Good Ol' Health Savings Accounts

In 1981 at what was then called the Executive Office Building of the Reagan White House, John McClaughry and I conceived the Medical Savings Account, later known as the Health Savings Account. John was at that time Senior Policy Advisor for Food and Agriculture, but he had read my book *The Hospital That Ate Chicago*, and it inspired him to think about a better way of financing health care. He asked me to come down to Washington to discuss the issue. We met and fleshed out the idea. Little did we then suspect how many delightful features would pour out of the simple little invention with only two moving parts.

It was patterned after the tax-deductible IRA (Individual Retirement Account) which Senator Bill Roth of Delaware was bringing out the following year. But with two major variations: our account contained the unique feature of a second tax exemption, given on condition the withdrawal was spent on health care. Otherwise, a regular IRA subscriber pays the usual income tax on withdrawals, and gets only one tax deduction, the one he gets when he deposits money into the account. Bill Roth later produced his second kind, the Roth IRA, which allowed a tax-exempt withdrawal, but took away the tax-exempt deposit. Only the Health Savings Account gives you both. In Canada, by the way, they do allow both deductions in their IRA, but in America only the HSA offers it.

Garlands of Unexpected Good Features. So **the first part** of a Health Savings Account is just that, a tax-exempt savings account, obtainable in the same way you get an IRA or a Roth IRA, although a few eligible outlets were slow to take ours up. And the **second combined feature** was to require a high-deductible, "catastrophic", stop-loss health insurance policy – the higher the deductible, the cheaper the premium gets.

Further, the more you deposit in the account, the higher is the deductible you can afford, so you save money going either way, and get extra benefit in your account for having a tailor-made insurance program. The industry term for this kind of insurance is "excess major medical", which the two of us wanted to avoid because of its implication it was somehow frivolous or unnecessary, when in fact it is central to the whole idea. Linked together, the two parts enhanced each other and produced results beyond the power of either, alone. The savings account was first envisioned to cover the deductible, but nowadays it also commonly attaches a special debit card to purchase relatively inexpensive outpatient and prescription costs. That led to further administrative savings to the subscriber if he shopped frugally for optimum proportions of deductible insurance. Right now, it's a little uncertain what the current Administration will permit in the way of catastrophic health insurance, so unfortunately it is just about impossible to give concrete examples of what the ultimate cost will prove to be. But we do know that in the old days, a $25,000 deductible was available for $100 a year. Nowadays, a $1000 premium is more likely. When we get to explaining first year and last year of life insurance, it will become clear that this premium can be appreciably reduced.

But while the savings account allowed someone to keep personal savings for himself, the insurance spreads the risk of an occasional heavy medical expense at what ought to be a bargain price for bare-bones insurance. You needn't spread any risk for small expenses because you control them yourself, but no one can afford some of those occasional whopper expenses. There's no reason why you couldn't set the deductible level yourself, weighing your own ability to withstand bigger risks. In practice, the actual savings were reported to approach 30% (compared with "First-dollar" health insurance), quite a pleasant surprise. But because of the younger age group of the early adopters, much of this saving was achieved in the out-patient area.

(Let's start using the present tense to talk about it, although right now it's hard to know what politics will permit.) So, hidden in this bland dual package are lower premiums, less administrative red tape, less moral hazard, but complete coverage. Right now, that's somewhat subject to change. It provides complete coverage in the sense that the insurance deductible can be covered by the savings account, but contains the option to be saved, invested or used for small outpatient expenses. Furthermore, the account carries over from year to year and employer to employer. So it eliminates job-lock, use-it-or-lose annoyances, and allows a healthy young person to save for his sickly old age. Curiously, many of the subscribers have elected to pay small expenses out of pocket, in order to make the tax deduction stretch farther.

In one deceptively simple feature, many of the drawbacks of conventional health insurance have been removed. The bank statement from the debit card can even do the bookkeeping. The first part of the two-part package, the savings account, creates portability between employers, opens up the possibility of compound interest on unused premiums, eliminates pre-existing conditions even as a concept, and creates a vehicle for transferring the value of being a "young invincible" forward into age ranges when the money really is likely to be needed for healthcare. Maybe some other features can be added later, but introducing an unfamiliar product is always greatly assisted by having it all appear so simple. The HSA only has two features, but they solve a dozen pre-existing problems.

To return to its history, nearly 15 million accounts have been opened, containing $24 billion. John McClaughry and I (neither of us received a penny for any part of this) were seeking a way to provide a tax exemption to match the one which employees of big business get when the employer buys insurance for them. That is, Henry Kaiser inspired us to do it. Although we got the general tax-free savings idea from Bill Roth, we did him one better by giving a deduction at both ends, provided only – you must spend the money on healthcare to get the second tax relief. An additional novelty at that time was a high deductible, which permits a "share the risk" feature unique to all insurance, but invisibly limits it to expensive items. It wasn't the original idea, but it turns out you get spread-the-risk and limits to out-of-pocket patient costs in the same package. Who could have guessed?

Volume control versus Price Control in Helpless Patients. We did know a third automatic advantage, not fully exploited so far: it seems possible the hateful DRG system (with its codes restructured) could become a useful tool for dealing with a major flaw in the Medicare system. Professional peer review has become pretty good at controlling the *volume* of services, but *prices* still escape effective control. No amount of volume control can, alone, address the price issue. Controlling vital services for helpless people is a delicate matter.

Quite a few of those services match (or contain) identical items in the outpatient area. The outpatient area faces outside competition from other hospitals, drugstores or vendors. Instead of letting helpless inpatients generate unlimited prices for the outpatients, why not let competition in the outpatient area define standards of prices for inpatient captives? Outpatients and inpatients overlap in the ingredient components, considerably more than most people suppose. Inpatients may have higher overhead because of the need to supply their needs at all hours, but a standard extra markup around 10% ought to take care of that. No doubt some services are unique to the inpatient area, but a relative value scale is then easily constructed, thereby linking unique costs to other services which are exposed to competition. Ultimately, provable relationships to market prices might even discipline big payers demanding unwarranted discounts. This last is a deal breaker, provoking suspicions of abused power by a fiduciary. Government in the form of Medicaid, is often the worst offender, so we need not imagine laws will prevent discounts so long as law enforcement remains crippled. Every business school teaches that discounts below cost are a path to bankruptcy, but business schools have apparently not had enough experience with governments to suggest an effective remedy.

Other than two variations (double tax deductions, and incentives if used for health care), a Roth IRA would be nearly the same as an HSA, with independently purchased Catastrophic backup. But the assured presence of low-cost, high-deductible insurance provides security for another needed feature :

> *"People end their lives with sickness, or else they must pay for protracted old age."*

Using individual accounts **with year-to-year rollover**, we could introduce the notion of frugal young people pre-paying the healthcare costs of their own old age. For all we knew, there weren't any frugal young people, but we were certainly pleasantly surprised. And catastrophic insurance added the ability to share the opportunity of that feature – subsidizing the poor at bearable prices. As we will shortly see, it also offers an incentive to save for retirement. Think of it: almost nobody can afford a million-dollar medical bill, but almost everybody welcomes low premiums. Catastrophic coverage offers the only chance I know, of approaching both goals at once. And it offers the fall-back, that if you are lucky and don't get sick, you can use if for your retirement.

As the only physician in the room, I also pointed out another pretty gruesome fact: either people end their lives having a lot of sickness, or they end up paying for a protracted old age. Only infrequently, do real people encounter both problems. It can happen of course; breaking a hip after a long confinement in bed would be an example.

Still More Good Features. Including these self-canceling needs in a single package allowed some flexibility between them – something badly needed for a century. We cannot go on passing a new regulation for every quirk of fate; a good program must allow some latitude.

Extended longevity tends to be hereditary, and so separate policies (sickness care and long-term care) are more expensive individually than the two combined, because the patient can out-guess an insurance company. Health Savings Accounts balance an incentive to save for one's own future health costs "at the front end" with reasonable cost limitations "at the time of later service", even though two time periods are decades apart. That's obviously superior to increasing the sickness subsidy at the back end, because, among other things, the patient will later have even more clues about his impending future. If cost reduction goes too far at either end, it amounts to an incentive to spend carelessly. Saving becomes fruitless.

A tax deduction is a tax deduction, but this one has two: An incentive to save, and a later option to spend the savings on either healthcare or retirement. That's nearly specific enough. Furthermore, it offers a choice between saving preferences – you can have interest-bearing savings accounts, or you can invest in the stock market, or a mixture of both. The HSA automatically converts to a regular IRA (for retirement) at age 66 when Medicare appears; that should be optional for all health insurance, but isn't. The IRA up in Canada includes both front and back features, but in the United States the HSA is the only savings vehicle to have dual deductions, so it's more flexible. As the finances of Medicare become shaky, it may be time to provide additional alternatives. At least, we ought to consider extending age 66 to a lifetime coverage option.

This harnessing of two familiar approaches makes a deceptively simple package which ought to be considered in other environments, unconnected with medical care. In most public policy proposals, the deeper you dig, the more problems you turn up. In this one, we found the proposal already had hidden answers to most concerns we could discover. It's possible to fall in love with an idea that does that for you. It lets you sleep at night, secure in the knowledge you aren't mucking things up for people.

Another surprise. Overall, the Affordable Care Act has probably helped sales of HSAs, since all four "metal" plans of the ACA contain high deductibles, serving in a (rather over-priced) Catastrophic role. This may be a way of covering the bets in a confused situation. The ACA is a needlessly expensive way to get high-deductible coverage, because it pays for so many subsidies. Frankly, it baffles me why subsidies swamp the costs of Obamacare, but are made unworkable for HSAs. Many of the details of the subsidies are obscure, including their constitutionality, so we have to set this aside for the moment.

One good motto is don't knock the competition, but we must comment on a few things. The Bronze plan is the cheapest, therefore the best choice for those who choose to go this way. But uncomplicated, plain, indemnity high-deductible, would be even cheaper if its status got clarified. The good part is, current rapid spread of high deductibles suggests mandatory-coverage laws may, in time, slowly go away. At first, the ACA looked like a bundle of mandatory coverages, all made mandatory at once. But they may be learning a few basic lessons as they go. Mandatory benefits are an example of mixing fixed indemnity with service benefits, with the usual dangerous outcome. Like many dual-option systems, they create loopholes. The HSA seems to avoid this issue by effectively being two semi-independent plans, for two separate constituencies – who are the same people at different ages. Once more, we didn't think of it, the features just emerged from the plan.

That's about as concise a summary of Health Savings Accounts as can be made without getting short of breath. But of course there is more to it, particularly as it affects the poor. For example, there is an annual limit to deposits in the Health Savings Account of $3350 per person, and further deposits may not be added after age 65. They can be "rolled over" into regular HSAs when the individual gets Medicare coverage, and supposedly has no further financial needs. So plenty of people have health care, but can barely support their retirement. These plans are absolutely not exclusively attractive to rich people, but it must be admitted, poor people start with such small accounts that companies can't operate profitably unless the client sticks with them for a long time. If people possibly can, they should scrape together one $3300 maximum payment to get a running start.

The problems of poor people can nevertheless be eased, within the limits of the plan's design. Since people will be of different ages when they start an HSA, it might be better to set lifetime limits, or possibly five-year limits, to deposits, rather than yearly ones. Some occupations have great volatility in earnings, and sometimes a health problem is the cause of it. To reduce gaming the system, perhaps the individual should be permitted to choose between yearly and multi-year limits, but not use both simultaneously. As long as the self-employed are discriminated against in tax exemptions, that point could certainly be modified. There remains only one major flaw, which we propose should be fixed:

> **Proposal 6:** Congress should permit the individual's HSA-associated Catastrophic health insurance premiums to be paid, tax-exempt, by Health Savings Accounts, until such time as elimination of the present tax exemption for employer-based insurance is accomplished by other means.

Subsidies for the Poor? Here's my position. If poor people could get subsidies for HSA to the same degree the Affordable Care Act subsidizes them, Health Savings Accounts should prove at least as popular with poor people as the Administration plan. Mixing the private sector with the public one is always difficult. Why not make subsidies independent of the health programs? There is no point in having the poor suffer because someone prefers a different health system. Quite often, a subsidy program is mixed with a public program, in order to make its passage more attractive; that's not necessary.

> **Proposal 7:** That health care subsidies be assigned to patients who need them, rather than attached specifically to one or another health system that happens to serve them.

Let's just skip away from all those digressions, and return to the poor in other sections. If the concern is, health care is too expensive, why in the world wouldn't everyone favor the cheapest plan around? Part of the answer, politics aside, is that young people have comparatively little illness cost, while old folks have a lot. Since Medicare therefore skims off the most expensive healthcare segment of the population, the fairness of any health subsidy program is difficult to assess. Evening out the tax deduction for the catastrophic portion equalizes the unfair tax deduction for self-employed and unemployed people. Perhaps the equality issue should be re-examined after each major revision, since many moving parts get jostled, every time.

The government is going to have trouble affording the existing subsidy, so it may not endure, particularly at 400% of the current poverty level. But if we can subsidize one plan, we can subsidize the other, instead. The government would then be seen, and given credit for, saving a great deal – by inducing destitute people to use HSA as an alternative option, equally subsidized by an independent subsidy agency. As for single-payer, the government for fifty years borrowed to continue Medicare deficit financing, and got it to 50% universal subsidy without much notice. That's like boiling the frog too gradually to be noticed, until it is too late. But suddenly expanding the 50% subsidy to the whole country at once, would definitely be noticed. Extending such levels to the whole country should anyway be buttressed with accurate cost data. Administrative cost savings are just a smoke screen. Total costs are the real cost. Other people also point out Medicare was financed after we had won some wars, but now we seem to be losing wars.

Simplified Math

L et's do some simplified math. The ancient Greeks, possibly Aristotle, discovered that money at 7% interest will double in ten years. By remembering this simple accident, you can follow the math of Health Savings Account in your head, without writing anything down. If you remember that life expectancy is now 84 years, you have eight, going on nine, opportunities to double your money. Go ahead and do it: 2, 4, 8, 16, 32, 64, 128, 256, 512, 1024. At the rate things are going, a dollar at birth becomes 512 dollars at age 90, and it isn't unreasonable to hope for a thousand-fold increase in the future.

The current expectation is an average of $350,000 in lifetime healthcare costs per person. A gift to the newborn of $350 will almost pay for it. If he sets this aside for a lifetime, forgets he has it, or just doesn't spend it, it will cover his costs. Medicare is about half of the lifetime cost, so $175 at birth would pay for a buy-out. The individual is already paying a quarter of Medicare as payroll deduction, and another quarter as premiums. So, it would cost something like $87.50

at birth to pay for the rest. Whether it's a gift of his family or a government subsidy, that is manageable. It's close, but it's manageable.

How do we get 7% interest? We assume an index fund of the total stock market will produce 11% per year, because that's what it produced for the past century, in spite of wars and recessions. We assume 3% inflation, for the same reason, leaving 8% net return. Because every 28 years on average we have a "black swan" stockmarket crash of 30-50%, you have to ride it out. Therefore, the conventional advice is to invest 60% in stocks and 40% in bonds, reducing your net return to 5%. But unlike a college or a museum, we have no payroll to meet, so we only use 60/40 after the age of 50, when major illness costs begin. That brings us up to 6.5% overall, after the HSA gets past its early transition costs. Since index fund investing is now readily available for less than a tenth of a percent management cost, we ignore the present fees of ten times that, which are customary. If you are forced to it, just put the certificate in your bank lockbox and have it opened when you die.

How much you actually invest at birth, or whether some other payment method is employed, are political decisions. The point to be made right now, is that passive investing of this sort is close to being feasible. It is close, but a cure for cancer or diabetes might make it a sure thing. The points to be made are two:

1. Adopting this approach with the Classical Health Savings Account, may or may not pay for the whole health system for everybody, but it would pay for a mighty big chunk of it.

2. The rest of this book, attempts to find a few other improvements which really would pay for the whole system with some confidence. There's no way to prove it was successful except to conduct some pilot programs. I would expect that dozens if not hundreds of other people would try to find other refinements.

Almost Good Enough

T hat's the good side of C-HSA. What continued to bother me was it was close to providing lifetime healthcare financing, but without much latitude. Perhaps it would be better to settle for half, or a quarter, which would

> *"Whole-life insurance is more profitable than term insurance, but it requires more capital."*

certainly have plenty of latitude for revenue shortfalls. Better still, perhaps a way could be found to phase it in, but stop when it runs low on money. Because it contained so many little pleasant surprises, however, I decided to press onward to see if others could be found.

What emerged were these new ideas:

1. Multi-year policies. To go from a term-insurance model to a whole-life model, using the life insurance approach. This would take advantage of the uptick of the yield curve in compound interest discovered by Aristotle long ago, inflecting at about the forty year mark. And advances in science would provide some extra years of longevity, to take advantage of it.

2. Escrowed Sub-Accounts. Instead of one big balance, it became apparent that some funds were intended for long-term use, and were therefore entitled to different interest rates (checking account, savings account, investment account), which the account manager would wish to have locked for a given time or purpose (66th birthday, ten-year certain, $10,000 minimum, etc.).

3. No age limitations. Further longevity could be introduced by making HSA a lifetime compounding experience, cradle to grave, but how to fund it remains an issue concentrated on the life alternatives facing those, age 21-66.

4. Birth and death insurance, catastrophic, disability, etc. Exploring the idea of HSA from birth, I came to realize the extra cost of the first year of life was a serious impediment to all pre-funded health schemes, since one can scarcely expect a newborn child to finance a debt of 3% of lifetime costs, in advance. To make matters worse, the

same is even true of the 8% of lifetime costs up to age 21. Thinking that one over, I came to see why nobody had ever devised a really adequate scheme for lifetime coverage. Seen in that light, it became clear the consequences justified solutions which might upset ancient viewpoints about a vital and sensitive subject. Whether recent turmoil (about same-sex marriage, unmarried mothers and the like,) would soften resistance or harden it, was just a guess. The result of this thinking was birth-and-death insurance, covering only the first and last years of life. Furthermore, it became easier to contemplate the issue of perpetuities, or inheritance from grandparent to grandchild. The laws already sanction inheritance to 21 years after the birth of the last living descendant, generally adequate for the purposes in mind here. All such special-needs insurance tends to reduce the remaining liability of general-purpose insurance, and typically is not workable unless the two insurers coordinate with each other and keep adequate records of their compacts.

5. Passive Investing and Dis-intermediation. The whole concept of "passive" index investing was borrowed from John Bogle of Vanguard and Burton Malkiel of Princeton. Recent difficulties in the fixed-income market make stocks seem just as safe as bonds to more people, and generally they provide more yield. The historical asset tables of Roger Ibottson of Yale inspired further confidence in the approach. Having absorbed this lesson, the concept of replacing an advisor with a safe deposit box emerged, although custodial accounts are not expensive. This maneuver could shift the "black swan" risk from the agent to the investor, assuming the agent has not shifted it, already. Ownership of common stock may not be entirely perpetual, but partial ownership of an index fund containing a trillion dollars worth of common stocks, certainly does seem perpetual enough for ordinary purposes.

6. Zero-balance protection devices. The potential that someone might figure out a way to game this system had to be considered, in view of the staggering magnitude of this proposed funding system if it caught on. The brake which suggested itself was to force the balances to return to zero at least once in a time period, and possibly many times oftener, if necessary. Offhand, I do not see how this system could be gamed, so the power to impose zero balances at a trigger level of balance, is a credible threat if it impends.

7. Total-market Index funds as a currency standard. One throw-away idea emerges from this analysis. The world economy went off the

gold standard some years ago, and since then has adjusted its currency by inflation targeting. In the recent credit crash, however, the Federal Reserve has been unable to reach the 2% goal for some time, for unknown reasons. If the reason for this remains unclear, or if the reason is unsatisfactory, it seems to me the total market index of the nation's common stock would be a superior proxy for re-basing the currency on the national economy. If other nations copied this standard, their central banks could agree on a system of leveraging it between currencies, but the essential fact would remain that each nation's currency was a proxy related to its national economy, ultimately based on the marketplace. That might even restore matters to where they stood before 1913, when the Federal Reserve was created. This certainly would be superior to what some people accuse the Federal Reserve of plotting (expunging our considerable debt to the Chinese by inflating our currency.) As people say, this matter is above my pay grade, but it certainly would have the advantage of stabilizing the medical system, and ultimately the retirement system. The need for protection against bit-coins might be kept in mind. If it prevented entitlements from off-the-books accounting, I would consider index funds as a currency standard, a considerable advance.

The addition of some or all of the above seven or eight features would provide more than enough extra money to fund the entire medical system until such time as it was forced, by scientific advances, to become a retirement fund with a small medical component. We have the rough estimate of $350,000 average lifetime medical cost, but no way at all of judging the average retirement cost, so this concept will have to terminate in fifty years or so, or when the data catches up with the theory. After all, the limit of desirable retirement income is not infinite for everybody, but it is obvious it is infinite for some people.

This synopsis of the additional concepts for Health Savings Accounts concentrates on paying for healthcare with a cash cushion in reserve, so it does not dwell on technicalities, favorable or unfavorable. It does however skip over one theoretical issue of some importance: where does this money come from? Linked to that is the wry observation that it proposes to reduce medical costs by spending gambling money from the stock market. Since people who would say that, show no reluctance to hurt my feelings, let me make a forceful reply.

The designers of the Medicare program in 1965 faced a huge transition problem, too, and nevertheless, plunged ahead in spite of badly underestimated future costs. So, although revenue surfaced in the HSA proposal had been there all along, it was never gathered and put to use – wasted, let us quietly say. I do not blame Wilbur Cohen or Bill Kissick for making concessions to get it started. There is little else they could do from 1965 to 1975 except adopt a "pay as you go" strategy. But sometime after 1975 that was no longer the case, and the new opportunity was neglected in a befuddled realization that costs were going to escalate rapidly, although hidden from sight. A great many free-loaders were added during the transition, and there was little to do except wait for them to die. So, yes, things were allowed to get worse than they needed to get, but as a nation we happened to be even luckier than we deserved to be, as scientists eliminated dozens of diseases we might have had to pay for. Until the end of that race between costs and revenues had come into sight, it was not possible to guess which one would win.

So now it is our turn to make proposals. We must face similar daunting problems of transition by a partially paid-up constituency, headed into a fully-expanded set of benefits for at least thirty years. Plus a huge and undeclared national debt from borrowing to pay for previous mistakes. I have tried to be generous in my assessment of the 1965 achievement, which was considerable. Let us see whether the opposition party can bring itself to respond generously and without intransigence, however vigorously they may subject the issue to adversary process. It doesn't mean to be a punishment, it means to be a rescue.

Investment Advice for Non-Investors

The cost of retirement living is probably already larger than the average lifetime cost of healthcare, or about $350,000. That's almost the same as saying nobody but a millionaire has a chance. But longevity is constantly lengthening, and healthcare will probably get cheaper eventually. So right now, retirement at $35,000 a year for 20 years is twice as expensive as healthcare, retirement at age 60 for 40 more years would cost four times as much as healthcare. Somewhere along the line, someone will suggest we make healthcare a minor component of retirement costs and roll the two together to save administrative costs. By that time, I expect healthcare to be largely an experience of retired people, anyway. With half the nation retired, the architects will have to design housing for that expectation. But the greatest challenge will be to find something for those people to do with their time. It might as well be – it almost has to be – something remunerative. Even assuming unlimited wealth, it's pretty hard to imagine people going on four ocean cruises a year, year after year. Or playing eighteen holes of golf, six days a week. I've known a few people who did things like that, but it's hard to imagine a whole nation doing it. And out of that synthesis will come some way to pay for retirement, including healthcare.

"Buy and Hold. Don't pay high fees. 6% Returns or Know the Reason."

The alternative is to have no money. Alternatives to watching television aren't attractive, and in fact they aren't much different from going to jail, except it is reported it costs more to be in Leavenworth than to go to Harvard. It's sixty or more years into the future, so it isn't my problem to re-design a civilization to fit its coming demography. All I can do is mention that having a regular check come in, won't be enough to occupy the time of half the country, so they better get started, developing something else. Meanwhile, here's how to arrange getting that check

For most of the past decade, saving for a rainy day has been in an interest-rate environment which made the usual saving process almost useless. Let's compare today with a generation ago. When my mother died at the age of 103, she had been living for decades on her savings account at the bank, with certificates of deposit and interest rates which were quite generous. She had a few stocks, but interest on fixed-income sources was the main thing, not just for her but for all the elderly folks in her generation. Well, for nearly a decade things have been entirely different for investors. The government has been trying to fight a recession with zero interest rates, and the Federal Reserve has accumulated trillions of dollars worth of bonds it will some day try to sell. Much of this has been financed artificially in ways most of us could not possibly understand, but we do understand two things:

1. A lot, if not most, of this maneuvering has been at the expense of old folks. They were taught to depend on fixed income, but interest rates right now are smaller than the rate of inflation, while the price of bonds has been driven high by the government owning trillions of them. They threaten to crash if things go back to normal, so somebody wants them to remain low. The Chairman of the Federal Reserve wants to be calm and reassuring, but essentially admits she isn't certain what to do.

2. When the Federal Reserve starts to raise interest rates back to normal, it will sell bonds, perhaps trillions of them. The bond market may not plummet immediately, but only if the Federal Reserve makes selling mistakes. Cash may be king in this situation, but only if investors don't freeze, like deer in the headlights.

So, It's a little hard to imagine buying bonds, living on bank accounts, or doing most of the other things we watched our parents do with great success. That would include Health Savings Accounts, wouldn't it? No, it wouldn't. The HSA is a good place to buy common stocks, and the best of all places to park your spare cash. You can invest in anything you please with HSA, with or without coupons, because a tax-free account doesn't care about tax consequences. If your HSA has any limitations to what you can do, it must be caused by your broker or your advisor, not because the HSA program gets in the way. Overfunding the HSA account is always a good alternative, although mostly a passive investment in a low-cost index fund of the entire American market will work out better. Let's put it this way: if you start investing when you are fairly young, you will probably come out well enough. If you start investing when you are nearing retirement age, you had better be lucky, because you won't have time to ride it out.

1. The first weapon you will have is compound interest. It has great power, because its secret is its effective interest rate rises at the far end. A small amount early in life is better than a big amount near the end, but any time is better than never. The tax exempt feature is a treasure. Thirty years extra longevity this century extend it longer, and longevity continues to increase. But remember this: the net income must be larger than the rate of inflation. If you don't know the rate of inflation, just guess it is 3% a year.

2. The second weapon is passive investing. Don't try to beat the market, just try to equal the market, and you will eventually get where you are going. But don't pay high fees. Lots of brokers have great track records until you subtract their fees. In fact, it is probably impossible to have a great record unless you charge low fees. Instead, buy an index fund of the entire U.S. Stock market, and act like you forgot you have it. And don't establish a Health Savings Account with the first agent you happen to meet. I once overheard my mother advising my daughter, "Don't marry the first man who asks you."

Some Unintended Opportunities

The present state of healthcare legislation is, to put it delicately, immature. Both Health Savings Accounts and the Affordable Care Act are the law of the land, but the Obama Administration defiantly slipped in some regulations, and quietly slipped in others, which have no precise authorization in the law. Everything may claim to be mandatory, but until enforcement begins, neither enforcement nor appeal to the Supreme

> *"By accident or by design, All Obamacare policy choices have high deductibles."*
> **The Bronze Plan is Cheapest**

Court about constitutionality seems completely feasible. When no one has been injured, no one has "standing" in the eyes of the courts.

Funding the Deductible. For example, every one of the governmental "metal" plans has at least a $1250 front-end deductible, going up to $6300 for full coverage. Meanwhile, non-government health insurance is rapidly replacing copay with high deductibles, too. (Co-pay is the main cause of supplemental insurance, a doubling of administrative burden.) Unless a person is eligible for subsidy, this mandatory large deductible makes the insurance hard to use unless the individual has saved up some cash for his deductible, somewhere else. So why not provide a tax incentive to have the deductible in escrow? At the moment, Health Savings Accounts are the only feasible approach to this goal, but that does not exactly mean they have been authorized to do so, since double coverage is more or less frowned upon. The deductible means nothing until you get sick, so Obamacare gave itself a few years to figure this out, but the public is apparently in jeopardy if it tries to invent a work around. It begins to look as though the voters may not give the originators of this plan enough time in office to see this as a problem they must address. So, if this is going to be everybody's problem, why not see if the Health Savings Account can offer to do it. By doing so, the individual apparently must drop his existing insurance, so go figure.

People who have no illnesses, naturally have little present concern with ambiguities in health insurance. But health insurance will matter as soon as illness appears. Therefore, the present state of limbo will increasingly be of concern to more people. Seemingly, there is a race between the three branches of government to start an action. Either a compromise must be reached between the Executive and Legislative branches, or else the Courts will be forced to intervene by some injured person. Curiously, the only Justice to express displeasure with the present Constitution is Ruth Ginsburg, whose two cancers make her likely to be the next Justice to retire.

A piggy-bank for Millennials. Whatever someone may think of Obamacare, the front-end deductibles provide a pretty substantial incentive to maintain at least $1250 per person cash reserve somewhere, and an HSA would be just a wonderful place to keep it. If that is somehow blocked, an IRA would be almost as satisfactory. If Congress addresses the matter, an IRA could later add a feature to roll over the deductible from such IRAs to HSAs. If the individual avoids spending what is in the HSA, it eventually will revert to an IRA on attaining Medicare eligibility, anyway. Calculating a 10% investment return, age 25, and assuming no medical expenses, it might then have grown to $51,000 taxable, or somewhat less if lower interest rates are assumed. For someone who stays healthy, its minimum distribution as an IRA at age 65 would start paying a taxable retirement income of over $775 a year. That's pretty good for an investment of $1250. Obviously, everybody older than 25 gets less, but in no case does anyone get less than the $1250 he/she put in, just to cover a possible deductible. The issue of the high investment return is taken up in Section Four. As will then be seen, there are two issues: whether such a return can be safe and consistent; and whether hidden fees will undermine the return.

It's true you can't spend the same money twice. If the fund is depleted by spending for a deductible, it must be promptly and fully replaced to keep the fund growing. However, Aetna studied and GAO confirmed, that only 50% of enrollees in employer-sponsored HRAs withdrew any of their funds (which might have been used for outpatient as well as high-deductible purposes). Apparently these clients were more anxious to preserve the tax shelter, than to protect their health, which is a slant I hadn't considered. This was true, even though the employers' efforts to enhance the compound income were not particularly strenuous. In a sense, it is a flattering sidelight on the frugality of many Americans. But the power of compound interest lies in re-investing the profits, so reasonably prompt restoration of the enhanced principal would not materially reduce the final outcome, just so long as internal profits remained untouched. It would be fairly simple to impose this requirement, creating a distinction between "balance" and "available balance", but doing things for people's own good, is always a questionable adventure.

We mentioned earlier, Roger G. Ibbotson, Professor of Finance at Yale School of Management has published a book with Rex A. Sinquefield called *Stocks, Bonds, Bills and Inflation*. It's a book of data, displaying the return of each major investment class since 1926, the first year enough data was available. A diversified portfolio of small stocks would have returned 12.5% from 1926 to 2014, about ninety years. A portfolio of large American companies would have returned 10.2% through a period including two major stock market crashes, a dozen small crashes, one or two World Wars hot and cold, and half a dozen smaller wars involving the USA. And even including one nuclear war, except it wasn't dropped on us. The total combined American stock market experience, large, medium and small, is not displayed by Ibbotson, but can be estimated as roughly yielding about 11% total return. Past experience is not a guarantee of future performance, but it's the best predictor anyone can use. The supply of small-cap stocks is probably a limiting factor. As we will see, your money earns 11%, but that isn't necessarily how much its owner will earn. But inflation throughout the period remained close to 3%. In this sense, the income net of inflation was never higher than 9%, so we have to presume 9% sets a theoretical limit to what can be achieved by passive investment, even after heroic efforts to reduce middle-man costs. Most of our estimates are based on 6.5%, and most investment managers produce less than that. Nevertheless, very substantial program gains are possible in every tenth of a percentage point which can be further squeezed out. The next candidate for streamlining cost is the Catastrophic insurance premium.

Catastrophic insurance has not been popular for many decades, so presumably there is room for competition to reduce premiums, marketing costs, profit margins, and other conventional competitive tools. The reimbursement to hospitals has suffered from favoritism directed toward some of its client corporation groups, who indirectly force Catastrophic to absorb some of their costs. And finally, there is likely to be overlapping provision for the same costs in a year-to-year system, which might be wrung out by five-year, ten-year or even lifetime policies. One can see potential economies on every side, but they will not come easily. In the long run, a perfect system might generate the revenue equivalent of 10.5% as a top limit instead of 9%. As everybody came up to speed, the potential is there for easily managing what might now be borderline achievable results. In fifteen years, that is. In the meantime, we will have to be satisfied with less ambitious projections for our present approach of term insurance.

So, in the meantime, we take things in a different direction, based on the whole-life insurance model. But one point may not be so clear: the Savings Account part of HSA is already lifetime, in the sense of rolling over and accumulating after-tax income for the rest of life. So for that matter, Catastrophic high-deductible insurance would be an easy next step, requiring only some adjustment of the present unfortunate tendency to assume an equivalence between "mandatory" and "exclusively mandatory". Money is money, and the courts will have to decide what sort of entirely fungible money is satisfactory for meeting minimum, maximum or any other coverage requirements. Since the "metals" plans all have high deductibles, but also have unduly high premiums, it seems likely the idea was to force insurance premiums to cover the subsidies for the uninsured. Such confusions of language and intent are ordinarily corrected by technical amendments.

At age 66, right as it now is, every HSA turns into an IRA for retirement purposes. But up until age 65 it can be used for medical expenses, getting a second tax deduction. We are close enough so that changes to enable a whole-life approach are imaginable, but not yet feasible.

Black Swans and Portfolio Content.

A standard deviation is the amount of deviation which is seen in two thirds of cases, and usually refers to the minor dips and bumps seen in a year. The standard deviation of the stock market in a year is about 2% – and can be ignored for this discussion. A much larger set of crashes occurs about once every thirty years, and is characterized by a crash of 30 to 50 percent. No one can afford to ignore something like that.

Protecting the investor against black swans is one of the few legitimate reasons for an investment return of less than 12%. Let's first look at how most big endowments handle the issue. A museum or university typically depends heavily on its endowment to keep it going. If it spent the full 12% of potential average endowment income in the good years, it might be unable to keep its door open during a black swan. It could set aside 30-50% of its endowment as a reserve for such contingencies, but income between recessions might go up to 15% and they would have missed it. A more conventional response has been to adjust the investment portfolio, so it maintains an annual investment return from a portfolio which is 60% stock, and 40% bonds. In the long run, that typically starts with a stock return of 12% and reduces it by a third to 8%, while investing the remaining third in bonds yielding 5%. Unfortunately, the long term experience is that inflation will nevertheless reduce all yields by 3%. So by prudent management of the endowment, a stockmarket yield of 12% is reduced to a spending rule of 5% (after inflation) representing what can safely be spent. Ouch!

> *"30% Dips, lasting several years, Every 28 years, on average."*
> **Black Swans**

Now, just a moment. We are talking about a Health Savings Account, not a university or an art museum. We aren't paying a big staff during hard times, we are investing for the far future, except for the fact the far future holds a different sort of terror for some, than for others. The young person may think he needs to pay his rent more than his drugstore bill. But he has so many years ahead of him, that may prove to be a very bad bargain, since depleting his account by a few hundred dollars may cost him thousands of dollars after he retires. If he can possibly borrow from his family, or reduce his college expenses right now, he should try to do it. A table should be prepared by his financial advisor at the HSA to convince him what is in his true best interests. It's a decision he should agonize over, not act on impulsively.

The converse is obviously true of a seventy year-old, choosing between a new car and Botox injections. Either one might be fine, but growing a fund he will never live to spend, is not so smart. And there are hundreds of situations between the two extremes. Here's one possible alternative, which straddles the issues:

Although the majority of situations vary from one extreme to the other in response to how old the person may be, financial managers often prefer solutions which tend toward one-size fits all because it creates a bigger pool, and maybe better returns. But it definitely wouldn't be wrong to get better returns for a little more risk. Especially for younger people when better returns cast a long shadow. Perhaps the portfolio should have a larger common stock content for clients up to age 50 than 60/40, perhaps 80/20 or even 90/10. The age of 50 is selected because health problems tend to increase after age 50. Or the ratio might be adjusted for the increased obstetrical costs of age 25-35, particularly for females. Actuaries should be consulted for more complicated issues. Since we definitely frown on kick-backs and other manipulations, perhaps fees should reflect the value of actuarial advice of this sort.

Expanding the Money in a Health Savings Account

L et's see how short and succinct we can make it. Our task is to take the maximum amount of savings we could possibly ask the public to accumulate, invest it more or less on autopilot, and see if it can generate enough money to pay for what we assume will be health costs a century from now. Some would say that's a fool's errand, but let's see what we can do.

We start with an assumption the average person can save $3350 per year from age 21 to age 66; that's $150,750, total, the most anyone can invest in an HSA. The actuaries at Michigan Blue Cross, verified by Medicare, estimate average life-time healthcare costs to be $350,000. Some people state you can stop

> *"Long Term Strategies."*

talking, right there, because that's too much money. Please be patient, we will address indigency later. For simplicity we wish to reduce the question to: whether we could turn $150,750 into $350,000 in forty-five years with compound interest at reasonable rates. The answer is yes. We can't predict whether those future predictions of costs are accurate, but if accurate, they can be achieved. We assume two things:

Indigents. We assume there will be no more indigents than at present. Can the government afford to subsidize them in this model? The answer is Yes, but its present commitment is in another direction, so it isn't entirely likely, very soon.

Outliving Your Income. We assume some people will use up their savings. If the average life expectancy, which is now 83, holds its present course, we assume this model can cope with it, even if the average life expectancy grows to be 93 in the next century. The arithmetic is quite favorable, but unfortunately we don't know what new costs will be added in the meantime. Assuming there are some, we aren't counting them, so predictions about the future all contain this flaw.

We assume some other things, mentioned as we go along, essentially coming to the conclusion the model will produce **a result which falls between the top and bottom curves in the graph.** Please note the narrow range of variation in the early years, and the widening upward range in later years. In particular, notice how a 3% (inflation) rate tends to stay flat well past any reasonable life expectancy, while more likely, investment income returns start to rise at age 60, and even sooner as the rate approaches 9% net of inflation. That seems to be a "sweet spot" the economy has discovered for itself in two hundred years of exploration.

We assume the equity stock market will follow the paths it followed since the Industrial Revolution. That is, it will produce an average of 12% gross return, with 3% of that eaten up by inflation, or 9% net of inflation. We then estimate our present conservative projections at producing at least 6.5% after costs, out of the remaining 9%. Dismissing inflation, we assume the stock market will operate between a 2% real return, and 9.5% real after inflation, leaving a 3.5% "cushion" for contingencies. When the Industrial Revolution ends, these basics may also change. We have a decade or so to try to get the investor's returns up closer to 8% safe level. And meanwhile, we must try to remain prepared for a bleak and bad depression, a "black swan", on average every 28 years, but individually unpredictable. In the meantime, we aspire eventually to pay for 100% of healthcare expenses, but <u>promise</u> to pay only a quarter of that. And finally, we assume medical care will change so much during the next century, that our calculations will need to be totally revised, long before then, with a so-called mid-course correction. With the understanding, that anything which pushes outside of the accompanying graph will have an obvious explanation, we assume future managers will make appropriate adjustments.

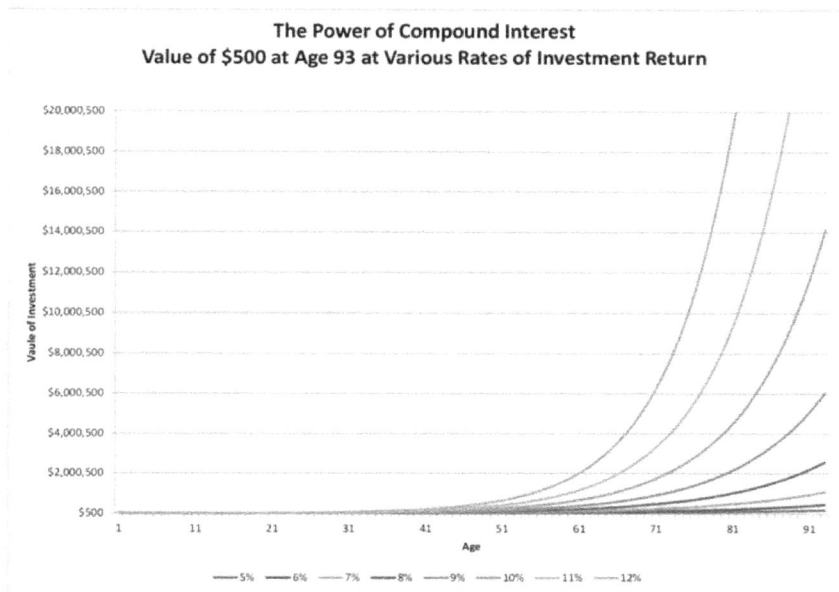

The Power of Compound Interest
Value of $500 at Age 93 at Various Rates of Investment Return

Single Premium Investment. Look carefully at the graph. It makes an unfamiliar assumption. It assumes a newborn baby started a Health Savings Account at birth, deposited $500 in it, and didn't touch the account again until he died. It is our assumption the average person could do that, perhaps with a stretch, and our further assumption that the government could do the same for indigent babies. There are times when neither the government nor many middle-class people could manage the necessary expenditures, but we set the value of $500 at birth as an extreme limit of what we think they both could do, on average most of the time. It's a number which is easily changed, if the economy varies from our projection.

Let's dramatize the point we're making on a totally different scale, by temporarily appointing Warren Buffett as its role model. According to a story in the Wall Street Journal by columnist Morgan Housel, this is the way the best investor in history made his money. At the age of eighty-four, his personal wealth was $73 billion. Of that, he made $70 billion <u>after</u> the age of sixty. Some might retort, the trick is to make the first $3 billion by the age of sixty, but a more civil underlying moral is that compound interest really starts to work toward the end of life.

Just take another look at that graph; the particular power of compound interest works as efficiently with $500 as with $3 billion. It starts earlier with higher interest rates, in this case age 40 at 12%, compared with age 85 at 5%, Mr. Buffett's numbers. Obviously, it pays to start early, and to get higher interest rates if you can do it safely. And conversely, it's a bad idea to spend or squander your savings while you are young. Our preferred method is to raise the interest rate by reducing the attrition of middle-men, in the approach mentioned earlier. You might not reach 12%, but you have a fair chance of reaching 9% if you allow yourself fifteen years to work on it. In the meantime, be satisfied with less than 100% coverage by this method.

More seriously, why else did we pick this way to depict the future? Because at age 66, when Medicare takes over, all of the plausible curves have reached a point where they could match Medicare's expenditures, indefinitely. If Medicare went broke, or was otherwise unacceptable for some reason, liquifying the account would produce a sum matching Medicare's present rate of expenditure. And finally, the numbers become so astronomical at the far end, it seems entirely reasonable to transfer part of the account to a grandchild's account. That trick alone should greatly reduce the problem, and add 21 years for compound interest to do it. As we will see in a coming section, paying childhood health expenses in advance solves some otherwise difficult issues.

Fun With Numbers

The principles of compound interest are thought to have been a product of Aristotle's mind. The principles of passive investing are more recent, mainly attributed to John Bogle of Vanguard, although Burton Malkiel of Princeton has a strong claim. In the present section, we propose to merge the two methodologies, compound interest with passive investing, trying to give the reader some idea why the combination could supply Health Savings Accounts with seriously augmented revenue. Because there is so much political flux, it cannot be an actual plan until the politically-controlled numbers have some finality to them.

The proposal to accumulate funds, however, shifts responsibility to the customer to spend wisely, even resorting to employing some of the individual's taxable money to pay small medical costs, thus preserving the tax shelter. (Or to use escrow accounts, or over-deposit in some other way, such as reducing final goals.) HSA doesn't directly reduce health costs, it eliminates some unnecessary ones, but provides lots of extra money to pay for essential ones. At the outset we want to state, schemes of this sort have a history of working effectively up to a certain level, and then begin to interfere with themselves as eager money rushes in. There's no sign of that so far, but it might appear. Therefore, we advise modest hedged experiments rather than attempts to pay for all of healthcare, reducing health costs perhaps by only a quarter or a half, since those smaller levels would still amount to large returns. Balancing the risks with investments outside the HSA – is just another prudent way of hedging the bet.

> *"Money earning seven percent will double in ten years."*

The rough rule of thumb is, money earning seven percent will double in ten years; money at ten percent will double in seven years. Seven in ten, or ten in seven. You can use simple maxims to verify the attached ideas. An early realization is that compound interest accelerates with time, and is highly sensitive to small interest rate changes. An improved rate of interest generated by (Twenty-First Century) passive investing gets multiplied by (Twentieth-Century) extended life expectancy. This idea might not have worked, a generation ago. And it will not work in the future, if future catastrophes shorten life expectancy, or interest rates rattle around. As happenstance, interest rates today rest near the "zero boundary", but interest risk is not totally eliminated. Interest rates have a way of bouncing, and irrational exuberance is part of our system.

In fact, we have a tragic example in the nation's pension funds. A few decades ago, pension managers were tempted to invest in stocks rather than bonds, and then the stock market crashed, stranding pensioners with low rates of return, rather than the high ones they had hoped for. I want readers to understand I am well aware of the cyclicity of markets, and make these suggestions, regardless. As long as we include a thirty-year "Black swan" contingency by limiting coverage to a quarter or a third, it should be reasonably safe, but savings would still be enormous. There are other, more traditional ways of protecting endowments from stock crashes. With people of every age to consider, the long transition period alone would almost automatically buffer out black swans.

Having issued a warning to be a conservative investor, let's now introduce some notes of reassurance. Younger people are always likely to be healthier. Those who save their money while young therefore need not use all of it for healthcare – for several decades. Compound interest works to magnify savings, the longer its horizon the better. We'll describe passive investing later, but it too should increase the average rate of return. These investments after some successes increase the incentives to save. If no one buys Health Savings Accounts, the incentives were apparently not large enough. If everyone rushes to buy, perhaps the incentives were unwisely too attractive. Right now, the financial industry is observing a rush to passive investing; nearly fifty percent of mutual fund investors are switching to "index funds" in spite of capital gains taxes on selling other holdings. Since the marvel of compound interest has been accepted for thousands of years, a mixture of compound interest and passive investing isn't an especially radical idea.

What's radical is the idea that all those highly-paid advisors can't do better than random coin-flippers. What's radical is to discover that a main ingredient of poor performance is high middle-man fees. Low fees won't assure high returns, but high fees will assuredly lead to low returns. If that new idea gets replaced in turn, it will be replaced by something better, and everyone should switch to it. But if compound interest is here to stay, this proposal is safer than it sounds. The investment income rate or continued employment of your agent are what isn't guaranteed, which is why **business relationships (between customers and managers of HSAs ought to remain portable and transparent by law**. Your manager might move, or you might decide to move away, from him.

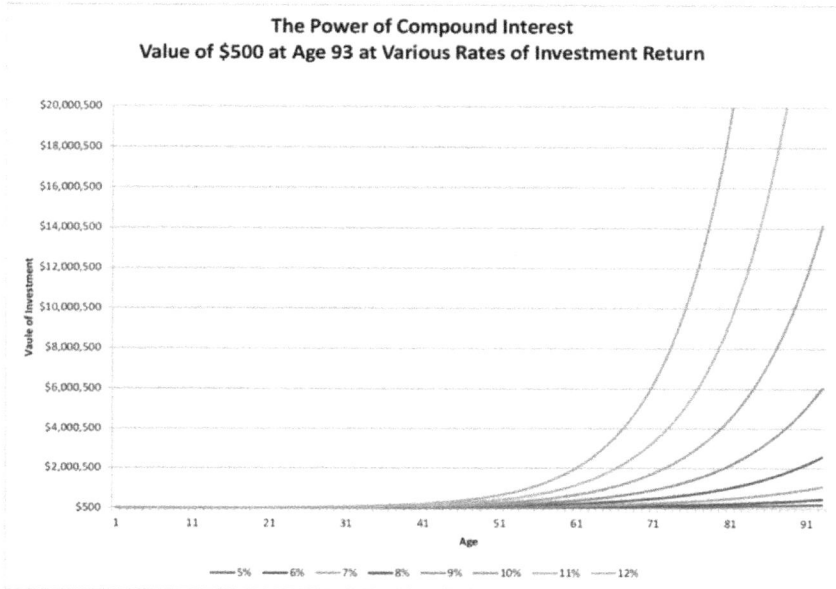

The Power of Compound Interest
Value of $500 at Age 93 at Various Rates of Investment Return

Start by looking at what happens if you jump your interest rate curve from 5% to 12%, or if you lengthen life expectancy from age 65 to age 93. That's what the graph is intended to show, and we stretch the limits to see what stress will do. Jumping to the highest rate (12%)the interest rate gets the balance to a couple million dollars pretty quickly, and lengthening the time period further enhances that gain. The combination of the two, easily escalates the investment far above twenty million. The combination of extra time and extra interest rate thus holds the promise of quite easily paying for a lengthening lifetime of medical care, regardless of inflation. In fact, it gets the calculation to giddy amounts so quickly it creates suspicion.

> *"Average lifetime health costs: $350,000 per lifetime."*

The actuaries at Michigan Blue Cross, verified by the Medicare agency, estimate average lifetime health costs to be around $350,000 per lifetime. That's just an educated guess, of course, but increasing interest rates and life expectancy will very easily surpass that minimum estimate. How do we go about it, and how far dare we go? Remember, our whole currency is based on the notion of the Federal Reserve "targeting" inflation at 2%, but in spite of spending trillions of dollars, they seem unable even to achieve more than 1.6%. We had better not count completely on schemes which require the Federal Reserve to target interest rates, because sometimes, they can't.

One person who does have practical control of the interest rate an investor receives, is his own broker. The broker shares the income, but usually takes the first cut of it, himself. Covering a full century, Roger Ibbotson has published the returns on various investments, and they don't vary a great deal. Common stock produces a return of between 10% and 12.7% in spite of wars and depressions; if you stand back a few feet, the graph is pretty close to a straight line. You wouldn't guess it was that high, would you? If you don't analyse carefully, a number of brokerages offer Health Savings Accounts which produce no interest at all – to the investor – for the first ten years. Indeed, income of 2% also amounts to nothing at all during a 2% inflation. In ten years, 2% approaches a haircut of nearly 20%, explained by the small size of the accounts, and by the fact that customers who know better will generally just politely look for another vendor. Since the number of accounts has quickly grown to be more than fifteen million, it might be time for some sort of consumer protection. The prospective future size of these accounts should command greater market power, quite soon. After all, passive investment should mainly involve the purchase of blocks of index funds, <u>all with fees of less than a tenth of a percent.</u> Much of this haircutting is explained by the uncertainties of introducing the Affordable Care Act during a recession, and taking six years just to get to the point of a Supreme Court Test, to see if its regulations are legal and workable. It can be used to provide high-deductible coverage, but it's expensive **That's the Theory.** The rest of this section is devoted to rearranging healthcare payments in ways which could – regardless of rough predictions – easily outdistance guesses about future health costs. When the mind-boggling effects are verified, sceptics are invited to cut them in half, or three quarters, and yet achieve a worthwhile result. The purpose here is not to construct a formula, but to demonstrate the power of an idea. Like all such proposals, this one has the power to turn us into children, playing with matches. By the way, borrowing money to pay bills will conversely only make the burden worse, as we experience with the current "Pay as you go" method. By reversing the borrowing approach we double the improvement from investment, in the sense we stop doing it one way, and also start doing the other. In the days when health insurance started, there was no other way possible. The reversal of this system has only recently become plausible, because life expectancy has recently increased so much, and passive investing has put that innovation within most people's reach. The environment has indeed changed, but don't take matters further than the new situation warrants.

Average life expectancy is now 83 years, was 47 in the year 1900; it would not be surprising if life expectancy reached 93 in another 93 years. The main uncertainty lies in our individual future attainment of average life expectancy, which we won't know, but probably could guess with a 10% error. When the future is thus so uncertain, we can display several examples at different levels, in order to keep reminding the reader that precision is neither possible, nor necessary, in order to reach many safe conclusions about the average future. Except for one unusual thing: this particular trick is likely to get even better in the future. Even so, it is best to do only conservative things with a radical idea.

Reduced to essentials for this purpose, today's average newborn is going to have 9.3 opportunities to double his money at seven percent return, and would have 13.3 doublings at ten percent. Notice the double-bump: as the interest rate increases, it doubles more often, *as well as* enjoying a higher rate. If you care, that's essentially why compound interest grows so unexpectedly fast. This widening will account for some very surprising results, and it largely creeps up on us, unawares. Because we don't know the precise longevity ahead, and we don't know the interest rate achievable, there is a widening variance between any two estimates. So wide, in fact, it is pointless to achieve precision. Whatever it is, it will be a lot.

Dollars at different Ages.

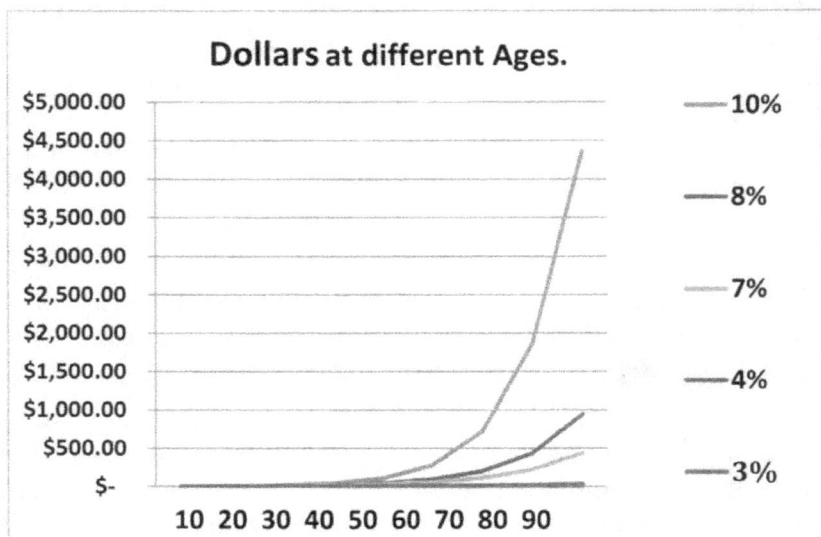

One Dollar: Lifetime Compound Interest

Start with a newborn, and give him a dollar. At age 93, he should end up with between $200 (@7%) and $10,000 (@10%), entirely dependent on the interest rate. That's a big swing. What it suggests is we should work very hard to raise that interest rate, even just a little bit, no matter how we intend to use the money when we are 93, to pay off accumulated lifetime healthcare debts. Don't let anyone tell you it doesn't matter whether interest rates are 7% or 12.7%, because it matters a lot. And by the way, don't kid yourself that a credit card charge doesn't matter if it is 12% or 6%. Call it greed if that pleases you; these "small" differences are profoundly important.

If that lesson has been absorbed, here's another:

In the last fifty or so years, American life expectancy has increased by thirty years. That's enough extra time for three extra doublings at seven percent, right? So, 2, 4, 8. Whatever amount of money the average person would have had when he died in 1900, is now expected to be eight times as much when he now dies thirty years later in life. And even if he loses half of it in some stock market crash, he will still retain four times as much as he formerly would have had at the earlier death date. The reason increased longevity might rescue us from our own improvidence, is the doubling rate starts soaring upward at about the time it gets extended by improved longevity. In particular, look at the family of curves. Its yield turns sharply upward for interest rates between 5% and 10%, and every extra tenth of a percent boosts it appreciably.

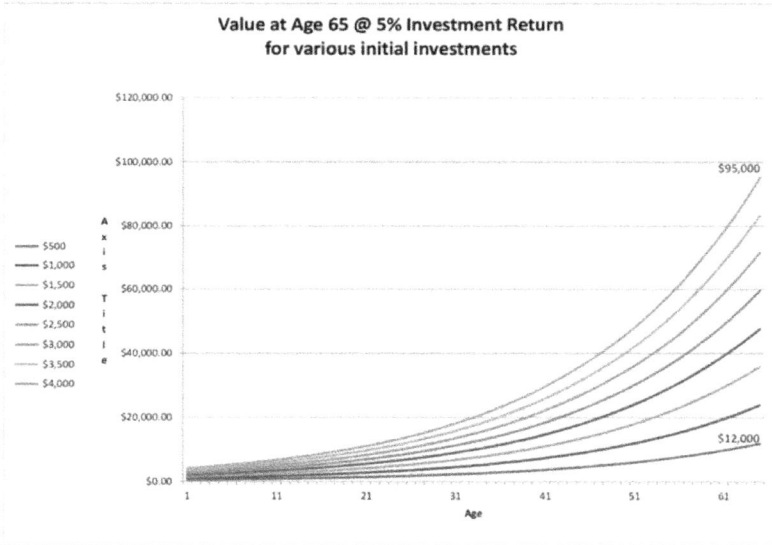

Value at Age 65 @ 5% Investment Return for various initial investments

Now, hear this. In the past century, inflation has averaged 3%, and small-capitalization common stock averaged 12.7%, give or take 3%, or one standard deviation (One standard deviation includes 2/3 of all the variation in a year.) Some people advocate continuing with 3% inflation, many do not. The bottom line: many things have changed, in health, in longevity, and in stock market transaction costs. Those things may have seemed to change very little, but with the simple multipliers we have pointed out, conclusions become appreciably magnified. Meanwhile, the Federal Reserve Chairman says she is targeting an annual inflation rate of 2% of the money in circulation; the actual increase in the past century was 3%. If you do nothing at 3%, your money will be all gone in thirty-three years. If you stay in cash at 2%, it will take fifty years to be all gone.

But if you work at things just a little, you can take advantage of the progressive widening of two curves: three percent for inflation stays pretty flat, but seven percent for investment income starts to soar. Up to 7%, there is a reasonable choice between stocks and bonds; but if you need more than 7% you must invest in stocks. Future inflation and future stock returns may remain at 3 and 7, forever, or they may get tinkered with. But the 3% and 7% curves are getting further apart with every year of increasing longevity. Some people will get lucky or take inordinate risks, and for them the 10% investment curve might widen from a 3% inflation curve, a whole lot faster. But every single tenth of a percent net improvement, will cast a long shadow.

But never, ever forget the reverse: a 7% investment rate will grow vastly faster than 4% will, but if people allow this windfall to be taxed or swindled, the proposal you are reading will fall far short of its promise. Our economy operates between a relatively flat 3% and a sharply rising 4-5%. In other words, it wouldn't have to rise much above 3% inflation rate to be starting to spiral out of control. Our Federal Reserve is well aware of this, the public less so. A sudden international economic tidal wave could easily push inflation out of control, in our country just as much as Greece or Portugal. On the other hand, as developing nations grow more prosperous, our Federal Reserve will control a progressively smaller proportion of international currency. Therefore, we would be able to do less to stem a crisis than we have done in the past.

To summarize, on the revenue side of the ledger, we note the arithmetic that a single deposit of about $55 in a Health Savings Account in 1923 might have grown to about $350,000 by today, in year 2015, because the stock market did achieve more than 10% return. There is considerable attractiveness to the alternative of extending HSA limits down to the age of birth, and up to the date of death. It's really up to Congress to do it. If the past century's market had grown at merely 6.5% instead of 10%, the $55 would now only be $18,000, so we would already be past the tipping point on rates. In plain language, by using a 10% example, $55 could have reached the sum now presently thought by statisticians – to be the total health expenditure for a lifetime. By achieving 6.5% return, however, the same investment would have fallen short of enough money for the purpose. Like the municipalities that gambled on their pension fund returns, that sort of trap must be avoided. Things are not entirely hopeless, because 6.5% would remain adequate if our hypothetical newborn had started with $100, still within a conceivable range for subsidies. But the point to be made, provides only a razor-thin margin between buying a Rolls Royce, and buying a motorbike. If you get it right on interest rates and longevity, the cost of the purchase is relatively insignificant. That's the central point of the first two graphs. For some people, it would inevitably lead to investing nothing at all, for personal reasons. Some of the poor will have to be subsidized, some of the timid will have to be prodded. This is more of a research problem than you would guess: a round-about approach is to eliminate the diseases which cost so much, choosing between different paths of research to do it, or rationing to do it. Right now we have a choice; if we delay, the only remaining choice would be rationing.

Commentary. *This discussion is, again, mainly to show the reader the enormous power and complexity of compound interest, which most people under-appreciate, as well as the additional power added by extending life expectancy by thirty years this century, and the surprising boost of passive investment income toward 10% by financial transaction technology. Many conclusions can be drawn, including possibly the conclusion that this proposal leaves too narrow a margin of safety to pay for everything. The conclusion I prefer to reach is that this structure is almost good enough, but requires some additional innovation to be safe enough. That line of reasoning will be pursued in a later chapter.*

Revenue growing at 10% will rapidly grow faster than expenses at 3%. As experience has shown, it is next to impossible to switch health care to the public sector and still expect investment returns at private sector levels. Repayment of overseas debt does not affect actual domestic health expenditures, but it indirectly affects the value of the dollar, greatly. Without all its recognized weaknesses, a fairly safe description of present data would be that enormous savings in the healthcare system are possible, but only to the degree we contain next century's medical cost inflation closer to 2% than to 10%. The simplest way to retain revenue at 10% growth, on the other hand, is by anchoring the price to leading healthcare costs within the private sector. The hardest way to do it would be to try to achieve private sector profits, inside the public sector. This chapter describes a middle way. It's better than alternatives, perhaps, but not miraculous.

Cost, One of Two Basic Numbers. Blue Cross of Michigan and two federal agencies put their own data through a formula which created a hypothetical average subscriber's cost for a lifetime at today's prices. The agencies produced a lifetime cost estimate of around $300,000. That's not what we actually spent, because so much of medical care has changed, but at such a steady rate that it justifies the assumption it will continue into the next century. So, although the calculation comes closer to approximating the next century (than what was seen in the last century) it really provides no miraculous method to anticipate future changes in diseases or longevity, either. Inflation and investment returns are assumed to be level, and longevity is assumed to level off. So be warned. This Classical HSA proposal, particularly with merely an annual horizon, proposes a method to pay for a lot of otherwise unfunded medical care. The proposal to pay for all of it began to arise when its full revenue potential began to emerge, rather than the other way around. If a more ambitious Lifetime HSA proposal ever works in full, it has a better chance, but must expect decades of transition before it can. Perhaps that's just as well, considering the recent examples we have of being in too big a hurry. Rather surprisingly, the remaining problem appears merely a matter of 10-15% of revenue, but all such projection is fraught with uncertainty.

Revenue, The Other Problem. The foregoing describes where we got our number for future lifetime medical costs; someone else did it. Our other number is $150,750, which is our figure for average lifetime deposit in an HSA. It's the current limit ($3350 per year of working life) which the Congress applied to deposits in Health Savings Accounts. No doubt, the number was envisioned as the absolute limit of what the average person could afford, and as such seems entirely plausible. You'd have to be rich to afford more than that, and if you weren't rich, you would certainly struggle to afford so much. To summarize the process, the number amounts to a guess at what we can afford. If it turns out we can't afford it, this proposal must be supplemented, and the easiest expedient is to raise the contribution limits. Other alternatives are pretty drastic: to jettison one or two major expenses, like the repayment of our foreign debts for past deficits in healthcare entitlements, or the privatization of Medicare. Not privatizing Medicare sounds fine to most folks, but they probably haven't projected its coming deficits. It would leave us considerably short of paying for lifetime health costs for quite a long transition period, but it might be more politically palatable, like Greece leaving the Euro, than paying more. Almost anything seems better than sacrificing medical care quality, which to me is an unthinkable alternative, just when we were coming within sight of eliminating the diseases which require so much of it.

Escrow Accounts and Over-Depositing. The main unpredictable feature of these future projections is you can't predict when you will get sick and deplete the account. Money withdrawn early is much more damaging than money withdrawn late in the cycle. Catastrophic insurance will somewhat protect against this risk, but the safest approach is to use segregated, somewhat untouchable, escrow accounts for future heavy expenses. That, combined with deliberate over-depositing, is the safest approach. If Obamacare would settle down, it might serve that function, as well, but the political situation is pretty unsettled until large-group design is made final, and that seems to mean November 2016 at the earliest.

Eligible Health Expenses

B ack when Health Savings Accounts were started, just about anything you could buy in a drugstore was a healthcare expense. However, if you go into a drugstore today, especially a chain drugstore, you can buy ice cream cones, cosmetics, shaving equipment and so many other things, you have a little trouble finding the pharmacist. Therefore, a debit card receipt from a purchase of a drugstore item will cover many more things than the Health Savings Account originally contemplated.

"Eligible-item Debit Cards"

Evidently, a number of people exploited this loophole, and it isn't surprising the regulators responded with regulations. The drugstores could have responded by making debit cards only apply to eligible items, but many didn't. So now you need a prescription from a doctor for the item, and you are subject to a 20% fine if you use the accounts for a non-eligible service. Some congressman could devise a system which would serve the purpose without the red tape, and Congress might get rid of this nuisance on behalf of the (now) 14 million subscribers to HSA, and the already beleaguered clerks in the drugstores. Next thing you know, the medical supply stores will start selling ice cream cones, followed by more regulations to prevent such evasions. That's of course the problem with depending on the stores to give up the illicit sales, in preference to giving up the red tape.

Several websites have started broadcasting lists of eligible items, hoping you will buy such items from them over the Internet, and eventually competition will sort this out. Meanwhile, we have to advise you to check the websites before you shop.

Longevity, a Moving Target

In the last fifty or so years, American life expectancy has increased by thirty years, enough extra time for three extra doublings at seven percent. So, 2,4,8. Whatever money the average person would have had when he died in 1900, is now expected to be eight times as great, since he dies thirty years later in life. And even if he should lose half of it in some stock market crash, he will still retain four times as much as he formerly would have, at the earlier death date.

The lucky reason increased longevity might rescue us, is the doubling rate started soaring upward at about the time it got extended by improved longevity in 1900 (when life expectancy was 47). In particular, look below at the whole family of curves. Its yield turns increasingly upward for interest rates between 5% and 10%, and every extra tenth of a percent boosts it appreciably more. Let's take a small example. Why don't we invest everything in "small" capitalization companies? Because there aren't enough of them to support such a large diversion to a frozen account. We are therefore forced to concentrate in large capitalization corporations, yielding only 11%. A few tenths of a percent extra yield might be squeezed out of this

curiosity. Life expectancy is slowly but steadily lengthening. And so on. It's useful for the nation to realize that having everybody live longer is a good thing, just as long as too many extra people don't get sick with something expensive.

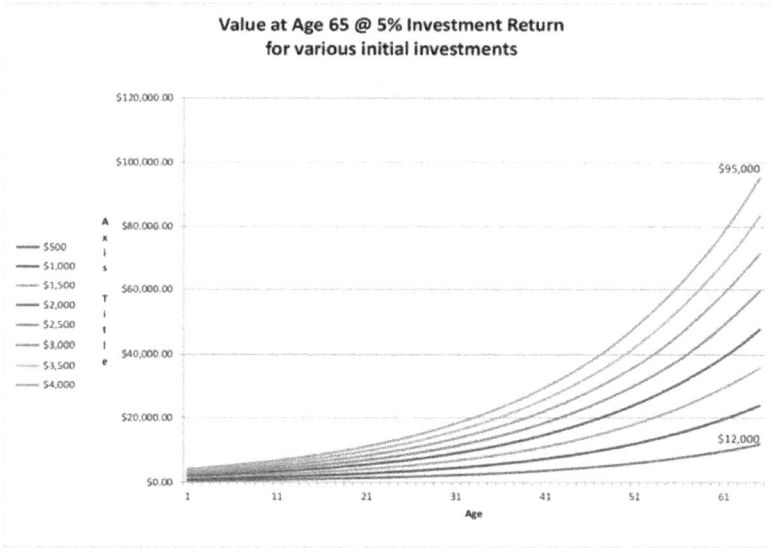

Value at Age 65 @ 5% Investment Return for various initial investments

In the past century, inflation has averaged 3% per year, and small-capitalization common stock averaged 12.7%. That results in an after-tax growth of 9.7%. Some people consider 3% inflation to be good for the economy, many do not. The bottom line: many things have changed, in health, in longevity, and in stock market transaction costs. Those things may have seemed to have deviated very little, but with the simple multipliers we have pointed out, that upturn in income at the end of life becomes steadily magnified. If you do nothing at 3%, your money will be all gone in thirty-three years. That is, if you leave your savings in cash. While it is true there are risks with all choices, the option of being a deer in the headlights is a poor one. There's a small but critical margin, and everyone must collectively struggle for very small improvements in it.

If you work at things just a little, you take advantage of the progressive widening of two curves, also shown on the graph: three percent (for inflation) remains pretty flat, but seven percent (for investment

155

income) starts to soar much earlier. Up to 7%, there is a reasonable choice between stocks and bonds; but if you need more than 7% you must invest in stocks. Future inflation and future stock returns may remain at 3 and 7, forever, or they may get tinkered with. But the 3% and 7% curves right now are getting further apart with every year of increasing longevity. Some people will get lucky or take inordinate risks, and for them the 10% (large-company stocks) investment curve might widen from a 3% inflation curve a whole lot faster. But except for desperate gamblers, every single tenth of a percent net improvement, will cast a long shadow. That means blue-chip common stocks are best, except during a black swan crash where all bets are off, but bonds are probably least bad.

> *"Save it, or Spend it. You can't do both."*

But never forget the reverse: a 7% investment rate will certainly grow much faster than 4% will, but if people allow this windfall to be taxed, gambled or swindled, the proposal you are reading will fall short of its promise. We are offering a way to minimize taxes, the other two risks are your own problem. Our economy operates between a relatively flat 3% and a sharply rising 4-5%. In other words, it wouldn't have to rise much above 3% inflation rate to be starting to spiral out of control. Our Federal Reserve is well aware of this, but the public isn't. A sudden international economic tidal wave could easily push inflation out of control, in our country just as much as Greece or Portugal if they leave the Euro. Another issue: As developing nations grow more prosperous, our Federal Reserve controls a progressively smaller proportion of international currency. Therefore, we could do less to stem a crisis than we have done in the past.

To summarize, on the revenue side of the ledger, we note the arithmetic that a single deposit of about $55 in a Health Savings Account in 1923 might have grown to about $350,000 by today, in year 2015, because the stock market did achieve more than 10% return. It might be more realistic to say $250 at birth rather than $55. but the principle is sound. You can't do it twice, but it ought to work, once. There is therefore considerable attractiveness to the expedient of extending HSA limits down to the age of birth, and up to the date of death. It's really up to Congress to do it.

If the past century's market had grown at merely 6.5% instead of 10%, the $55 would now only be $18,000, so we would already be past the tipping point on rates. You do have to leave some extra room. In plain language, by using a 10% example, $55 could have reached the sum now presently thought by statisticians – to be the total health expenditure for a lifetime. But by accepting 6.5% return, the same investment would have fallen well short of enough money for the purpose. Unlike the municipalities that gambled on their pension fund returns, that sort of trap must be anticipated to be avoided.

Things are not entirely hopeless, because 6.5% would remain adequate if our hypothetical newborn had started with $100, still within a conceivable range for subsidies for the poor. But the point to be made, provides only a razor-thin margin between buying a Rolls Royce, and buying a motorbike. If you get it right on interest rates and longevity, the cost of the purchase is relatively insignificant. That's the central point of the first two graphs. For some people, it would inevitably lead to investing nothing at all, for personality reasons. Some of the poor will have to be subsidized, some of the timid will have to be prodded.

This is more of a research problem than you would guess: a round-about approach is to eliminate first the diseases which cost so much, choosing between research to do it, or rationing to do it. Right now we have a choice; if we delay, the only remaining choice would be rationing.

> **Commentary.** *This discussion is, again, mainly to show the reader the enormous power and complexity of compound interest, which most people under-appreciate, as well as the additional power added through extending life expectancy by thirty years this century, and the surprising boost of passive investment income toward 10% by financial transaction technology. Many conclusions can be drawn, including possibly the conclusion that this proposal leaves too narrow a margin of safety to pay for everything. The conclusion I prefer to reach is that this structure is almost good enough, but requires some additional innovation to be safe enough. That line of reasoning will be pursued in a later chapter.*

Revenue growing at 7% will relentlessly grow faster than expenses at 3%. As experience has shown, it is next to impossible to switch health care to the public sector and still expect investment returns at private sector levels. Repayment of overseas debt does not affect actual domestic health expenditures, but it indirectly affects the value of the dollar, greatly. With all its recognized weaknesses, a fairly safe description of present data would be that enormous savings in the healthcare system are possible, but only to the degree we contain next century's medical cost inflation closer to 2% than to 10%. The simplest way to retain revenue at 7% growth is by anchoring the price leaders within the private sector. The hardest way to do it would be to try to achieve private sector profits, inside the public sector. This chapter describes a middle way. Better than alternatives, perhaps, but nothing miraculous.

What HSA Does for Poor Folks: A Proposal

When I give talks about Health Savings Accounts, there often seems to be some person in the front row who doesn't seem to be listening. But he's usually the first to raise his hand with a question, which goes more or less like this: **"Well, what does this do for poor people?"** So here's my usual answer.

Poor people are all poor, but they are poor in different ways. For preliminary discussion, let's divide them into three classes.

On Their Way Up. Most Americans came here at the bottom, and worked their way up. Poverty may once have been their condition, but it wasn't their ambition to stay there. Everyone, particularly the newcomers, can see that cheaper means more people can afford something they once couldn't afford. It's the job of Health Savings Accounts to make healthcare cheaper, but if you subsidize more than half of the population, and then set a threshold of 400% of poverty, you tend to hold people in place. You tend to make subsidies hard to surrender, which increases the number of subsidized people, and ultimately makes subsidies too expensive to continue. It may be well-intended, but it makes things worse. The Latin expression

"Like Tolstoy's Unhappy Families, Poor people are Poor in Different Ways."

Primum non nocere is the medical profession's motto, meaning "The least you can do for somebody, is not make their problem worse." On the other hand, by making healthcare cheaper, more people can afford it, so you've done a lot of good.

Stuck at the Bottom. It's true a dismaying number of people are permanently unemployable. Not just unemployed, but unemployable. The Mayor of my little suburb tells me 8% of the school budget is devoted to "Special education", which mostly means mental defects of one kind or another. In spite of special education, a large proportion of mentally retarded kids will never be able to support themselves. And despite movies about Nobel prize winners with Lou Gehrig's disease, a lot of other people born with neurological conditions will never be self-supporting, either. My profession is working hard to reduce the number of permanently disabled, and quite often it is fiercely expensive to treat them, but we keep doing it. For the most part, these disabilities are easy to recognize, and with few exceptions it is society's obligation to subsidize them indefinitely. But it is not the role of Health Savings Accounts to define, identify or treat these people. In fact, it would injure our performance to take on a non-financial role. Give us the money and we will expand it and then pass it along. We will even contribute toward its cost, but much prefer to have government pay its own bills, and not disguise their taxes as part of our operating budget. Who made it government's duty? Our elected representatives in Congress did, and we try to follow their rules.

Temporary, Borderline and Political. For a while, I acted as a referee on Disability Determination. Let me tell you, it's often pretty hard to tell who is malingering, from who is eligible among a host of different assistance agencies, and who has long since recovered from a disabling condition. It's therefore expensive to administer Disability Determination, and physically exhausting if you take it seriously. It isn't the proper job for a Health Savings Account, which would do it very poorly, dragging down the performance of what else we would really like to do perfectly. Which is to reduce the effective cost of healthcare, by adding an unexploited source of revenue in the financial field.

HSA Proposal for the Poor. The proposal, therefore, is we should start with what is least controversial in almost everybody's mind, which is catastrophic health insurance. This type of insurance comes closest to what everyone would agree we owe all our citizens. No money is expended on the basis of income or social circumstances, it is decided individually at the hospital door, usually by accident room physicians. Its volume of component services would be controlled by an improved DRG, and its retail price should be determined by outpatient costs determined in turn by the marketplace, or by a relative value scale when no comparable outpatient service exists. It may be advisable to reconstitute the PSRO (Professional Standards Review Organization).

It may be desirable to dispense this catastrophic insurance through an HSA, although it is not essential. If it is the only benefit provided, it still would be useful to provide an accordion mechanism for additional services for those who rise from poverty, who are reimbursed through special programs in a variety of ways, or who find ways to supplement the cost themselves. Ultimately, it should provide a vehicle for integration, temporarily or permanently, into the private sector.

Commentary: Agency for Mid-Course Corrections

Among the many things we don't know about the future, is the average longevity eighty years from now. The whole-life insurance industry prospered when they sold policies assuming American longevity of 47 years in year 1900, and it turns out to be 83 today, still growing fast. If longevity should get shorter, as it recently has in Russia, life insurance would go out of business. Since we can't rely on projections, we have to rely on early observations, and make mid-course corrections.

> *"So, who is counting."*
> **Quis custodiet custodies?**

President Lyndon Johnson both underestimated how much Medicare would cost, and how politically successful it would be. He was in no position to multiply 50 million Americans times $11,600 per year per person, times 22 years per person. That simple sentence tells you all you need to know about current Medicare costs, but who knew? Nor could he know how fast longevity would grow, or how fast the cost would rise. But we can monitor the trend, extrapolate, and revise the extrapolation. Medicare was a medical success, which had to be paid for; and President Johnson's successors might have found that out a little sooner, and changed course. If we must find fault, failure to readjust early, would be my candidate.

For reasons obvious or not, the nation would be well served to create a monitoring agency for the guidance of future Congresses in charge of the type of Health Savings Accounts we already do have, and maybe some related issues. When we start envisioning lifetime coverage, it becomes even more vital to have a permanent agency to sort out what is happening. This is particularly important when the Branches of the Federal Government are divided between the two parties. Informally, the subcommittees of the Appropriations Committees have assumed much of the burden of overseeing agencies. They are the only Congressional Committees to review every program every year. However, the Agencies have grown to be the largest bureaucracies in the government, and tend to become jealous of their independence, as the Appropriation Committees grow too burdened to bother with them. It begins to look as though we need more Congressmen if we want Congress to maintain a closer control of the agencies. Each Congressman now represents a million constituents, and simply cannot do all we would like him to do. As much as anything, we need a core group who worry about issues in advance, and have the prestige and access to make their views be heard. Rather than design a blueprint, let's review some issues that such a body might explore.

> **Proposal 8:** Health Savings Account Age Limits Should be Extended, from the Cradle to the Grave. A few extra years might be a minor improvement in special cases. The real benefit would be to create a continuous account, which could grow over long periods of apparent inactivity.

> **Proposal 9:** Instead of annual contribution limits, the limit for HSA should extend over several years, or even be a lifetime limit. When deposits must be skipped for health or occupational reasons, there should be an opportunity to catch up. Athletes and similar occupations tend to concentrate earning power in a few years.

Since the HSA is increasingly accustomed to augmented retirement income, thought should be given to extending the idea to amounts of money which could encourage that use. Furthermore, there are special circumstances, like a partial Medicare buyout, in which a limit to deposits forces a choice between two desirable uses for the same money. If the individual has the money for more than one purpose, it seems wrong to force a choice. For example, it's considerably safer to over-deposit more than you believe you will need, planning to return the excess. As a practical matter, the usual danger is overoptimistic revenue projection. Someone who sells his business at age 63 might have enough cash, but still encounter trouble with the $3300 per year limit because he once needed the income to run the business. It seems pointless to squeeze through such a narrow window, and much better if the window were at least enlarged to permit lump-sum deposits up to a $132,000 lifetime limit. With that sort of cushion, plus a stretch of reasonably good health at the right time of life, it would become considerably safer to take risks. At age 65, a lifetime of health costs is already in the past, but the curve of health expenses starts to bend upward at age 50, at a time when college expenses for children may be persisting, and the house isn't quite paid for. It seems a pity to cripple a good idea with pointless contribution limits that almost stretch far enough, but leave people fearful. If Congress develops a serious interest in lifetime insurance, the yearly contribution limit should be revisited. The optional side use for retirement should be examined in parallel, including its potential for being gamed.

Revisited by whom? Someone should be empowered to travel, and talk to people in the field. Maybe hold hearings, maybe just interview. A simplified goal is therefore to accumulate $80,000 in savings by the 65th birthday, intending to make a single-premium buy-out. That clarifies costs, but is it practical on a large scale?Remember that savings get a lot harder when earned income stops. With current law, you would have to wake up and start maximum annual depositing of $3300 by your 50th birthday, to reach $80,000 by age 65, and you would need generous internal compounding to make it. But notice how easily $100-200 a year would also get you there, starting at age 25 (see below), even justifying somewhat less optimistic investment income returns until age 65.

Many more frugal people might skin by with looser rules; It even could rather easily be subsidized for poor people and hardship cases. If you are going to cover lifetime health costs instead of just Medicare, many more will need $80,000 to do so, and have something left to share with the less fortunate. But to repeat once again, that still compares favorably with the $325,000 often cited as a lifetime cost. That's all we care to promise in public, but secretly we know it may not be enough. The plain fact is, if longevity or inflation get out of hand, someone must have the authority to raise the contribution limits, and to do that, there should be some research by a trusted house actuary.

> **Proposal 10:** Instead of the present annual limit of contributions to Health Savings Accounts of $3300 per year, Congress should permit a lifetime limit of $132,000, with annual deposit limits adjustable to bring accounts at their present age, up to what they would have been if $3300 annually had been deposited since age 25.

> **Proposal 11:** Congress should reserve decisions to itself for changing the lifetime contribution level, and review final appeals from contract terms which seem to threaten imminent major adjustment to the general public lifestyle

The Cost of Pre-funding Medicare. Rates of 10% compound income return would reduce the required contribution to $100 per year from age 25 to 65, but if the income were only 2% would require $700 contributed per year, and at 5% would require $300 per year. Remember, we are here only talking of funding Medicare, as a tangible national example.

It is this calculation, however rough, which has made me change my mind. It was my original supposition that multi-year premium investments would only apply up to age 65, and that would be followed by Medicare. In other words, HSA should only be implemented as a less expensive substitute for the Affordable Care Act. It seemed to me the average politician would be very reluctant to agitate retirees by proposing a plan to eliminate Medicare. They would feel threatened, the opposing party would then fan the flames of their fears, and the result would have a high likelihood of undermining the whole idea for any age group, for many years. Better, I thought, to take the safer route of avoiding Medicare, and confining the proposal to working people, where its economics are overwhelmingly favorable.

But when the calculations show how close this proposal under cautious revenue projections could come to failure, and when nothing else remotely close to it has been proposed by anyone, the opportunity runs the risk of passing us by. So, I have changed my mind. The moment of opportunity is too fleeting, and the consequences of missing it entirely are too close, to worry about the political disadvantage of doing the right thing. The transition to a pre-funded lifetime system will take a long time to get mature, and the political obstacle course preceding it is a daunting one. At least we should allow it as a demonstration option, where some fears will prove unwarranted, while others can be corrected.

So we make the guess of the average life expectancy where things will eventually flatten out, will then be about 91. (Be careful, most census figures are for life expectancy-at-birth.) But many people would have to be lucky in all details: a favorable investment climate for the right ten-year periods, plus a favorable health situation which avoids expensive illnesses just at the age when they begin to threaten. Some life-saving scientific advances would be a big help, too. Using a lower goal of $80,000 and an interest rate of 7% is considerably easier to conjure, but the barrier which might be reached first is the $3300 yearly contribution limit. Some unfortunate individuals might be forced to pay all medical expenses out of pocket in order to make the investment fund stretch, even before the average becomes affected. The individual who came up short might still remain considerably ahead of where he would be without an HSA, but we are using a precise match of revenue and expense, to simplify the examples.

Someone who sells his house or business at age 63 might have the cash, but still have trouble because of the $3300 per year deposit limit. It seems pointless to squeeze through a narrow window, and much better if the window were enlarged to permit lump-sum deposits up to a $132,000 lifetime limit, adjusted for inflation and compound income returns. With that sort of cushion, plus a stretch of reasonably good health at the right time of life, it would become considerably safer to take the risks. At age 65, a lifetime of health costs is nearly in the past, but the curve of health expenses starts to curve up at age 50, at a time when college expenses for children may be persisting, and the house isn't quite paid for. It seems a pity to cripple a good idea with pointless contribution limits that almost stretch far enough, but leave people fearful. If Congress develops a serious interest in lifetime insurance, the yearly contribution limit should be revisited.

The simplified goal is therefore to accumulate $80,000 in savings by the 65th birthday, remembering that savings get a lot harder when earned income stops. With current law, you would have to start maximum annual depositing of $3300 by your 50th birthday, to reach $80,000 by age 65, and you would still need generous internal compounding to make it. But notice how easily $100-200 a year would also get you there, starting at age 25 (see below) and less optimistic investment income returns until age 65. Many more frugal people might skin by with looser rules; poor people and hardship cases could more easily be subsidized. If you are going to cover lifetime health costs instead of just Medicare, many more will need $80,000 to do it, and have something left to share with the less fortunate. But to repeat once again, that still compares very favorably with the full $325,000 which is often cited as a lifetime cost. We have already imposed an extra $80,000 internal savings requirement in order to include Medicare; here is the place it would be a hardship. That's about as far as concentrated thought will carry you. It leads to the conclusion that it might be better to modularize Medicare and let the public pick and choose what it wants to buy its way out of.

The Cost of Pre-funding Medicare. Rates of 10% compound income return would reduce the required contribution to $100 per year from age 25 to 65, but if the investment income were only 2% would require $700 contributed per year, and at 5% would require $300 per year. Remember, we are here only talking of funding Medicare, as a well-understood national example, Obviously, a higher return would provide affordability to many more people than lesser returns. When $100 competes for the investment income from 10%, it's much easier than $300 competing for 5% income. Let's take the issues separately, but don't take preliminary numbers too literally. They are primarily intended to alert the reader to the enormous power of compound interest, and the big difference made by relatively small changes in it. Let's go forward with some equally amazing investment discoveries which are more recent, and vindicated less by logic than empirical results.

A transition from term insurance to pre-payment of Medicare is greatly eased by forgiving the premiums and payroll deductions, which are roughly age-distributed, and can therefore be forgiven in a graduated manner for late-comers to the program. Most cost-redistribution of high-cost outlier cases should be handled through the catastrophic insurance, which is well suited for invisible and tax-free redistribution. Because of hospital cost-shifting, inpatients are temporarily overpriced, but are quickly becoming underpriced as a result of hospitals gaming the DRG to shift costs to outpatients. This will in time affect the relative costs of Catastrophic and Health Savings Accounts, and must be carefully monitored for mid-course adjustments. This changing horizon of cost shifting reinforces the need to create a special agency to keep track of it. And to report its findings to Congress, who can consider the broader political implications, once they know the facts.

> **Proposal 12:** Congress should create and fund a permanent Health Savings Account Agency. It should have members representing subscribers and providers of these instruments, with power to hold hearings and make recommendations about technical changes. It should meet jointly with the Senate Finance Committee and the Health Subcommittee of Ways and Means periodically. It should have extensive access to the appropriate Executive Branch department, to review current activity, detect changing trends, and recommend changes in regulations and laws related to the subject. On a temporary basis, it should oversee inter-cohort and outlier loans, leading to recommendations about the size and scope of inter-subscriber loan activity. At first, it might conduct the loan activity itself, with an eye toward eventually overseeing a commercial vendor.

Cost Sharing with Frugality. At present costs, statisticians estimate future healthcare costs of about $325,000 (in year 2000 dollars) for the average lifetime. We could discuss the weaknesses of that estimate, but even though it's breathtaking, it's the best guess available. Women experience about 10% higher lifetime health costs than men. Roughly speaking, how much the average individual somehow has to accumulate, eventually must equal what he spends by the time of death. The dying individual himself has little interest in what is left unpaid at his death, so Society must do it for him, in order to survive as a Society. At this point, we unfortunately must also work around one of the great advantages of having separate accounts.

On the one hand, individual accounts do create an incentive to spend wisely, but it is also true that pooled insurance accounts make cost-sharing easier, almost invisible, and tax-free. Cost sharing induces reckless spending of other people's money however, while individual accounts induce frugality with your own money. Therefore, linking Health Savings Accounts with Catastrophic insurance provides a way to pool heavy outlier expenses, while the incentive for careful money management remains in the outpatient costs most commonly employed (together with a special bank debit card) to pay outpatient costs. Such expenses are much more suitable for bargain-hunting anyway, because dreadfully sick people in a hospital are in no position to argue or resist.

But a cautionary reminder: linking individual accounts to frugality through outpatients, as well as linking heedless spending to insurance through inpatients – induces hospital administration to game the system we have here imagined. There's no doubt a system can be gamed by shifting medical care to the outpatient area, but we must expect the DRG to be attacked, in order to reverse such incentives, which run in the hundreds of billions of dollars. A well-informed monitoring system simply must be created and funded, if we ever expect the decision to hospitalize patients to rest on whether the patient needs to lie down, instead of on what kind of payment system we happen to fancy. At the same time, the present DRG coding system must be considerably improved to withstand being subverted. These are not tasks which congressmen typically enjoy, but they must be done within the legislative branch if we expect it to function.

Standard Deviation within and between age cohorts. Furthermore, there is an important distinction between a mismatch of revenue to expenses caused by chance within one age group, and a revenue mismatch between two age cohorts. To put it another way, somebody has to pay off these debts, and we must have a plan about who should pay them when revenue is not present in the account. Borrowing between subscribers within the same age cohort should pay modest interest rates to forestall gaming, but borrowing between different cohorts for things characteristic of their age level (pregnancy, for example) should pay no interest if at all feasible. Unfortunately, people sometimes abuse such opportunities, and interest must then be charged. Until the frequency of such things becomes better established, this function of loan banking policy should be part of the function of the oversight body, rather than the executive agency, which tends to want to retain the function. When its limits become clearer, it might be delegated to a bank, or even privatized, but the policy must be monitored by specialists who understand what is happening "on the ground". While it is unnecessary to predict the last dime to be spent on the last day of life, incentives should be understood by the managing organization, separating routine cash shortages from likely abusive ones. And looking at all such activity as potentially having been caused by payment design. Much of this sort of thing can be minimized by encouraging people to over-deposit in their accounts, possibly paying some medical bills with after-tax money in order to build the fund up. Such incentives must be contrived, if they do not appear spontaneously. User groups can be very helpful in such situations. People over 65 (that is, those on Medicare) spend at least half of that $325,000 lifetime cash turnover, but just what should be counted as careless overspending, can be a matter of argument.

> **Proposal 13:** Current law permits an individual to deposit $3300 per year in a Health Savings Account, starting at age 25, and ending when Medicare coverage begins. Probably that amount is more than many young people can afford, so it would help if the rules were relaxed to roll-over leftover entitlements to later years, spreading the entire $132,000 over the forty-year time period at the discretion of the subscriber.

SECTION FOUR

New Health Savings Accounts

The project combines several concepts developed in other chapters, but is ready to be considered as a whole.

Introduction

Having so far described some of the nuts and bolts of Health Savings Accounts, we here sketch in a more specific variation which might be possible under various political circumstances. The original idea was to explore the problems, and potential solutions, attendant to avoiding age group 21-66, and seeing what could be done with the rest.

It turns out that working age people support the other age groups so heavily the two cannot safely stand alone. The funding advantage enjoyed by people 21 to 66 is weighted down by payroll deductions for Medicare, which are only half as large as the 50% government subsidy of Medicare. The overall effect destabilizes every age group. Only the 44% who are members of large employee groups are able to fund themselves, assisted by federal tax subsidies and local hospital discounts. The hidden Medicare deficit thereby threatens the whole system, and should have been addressed decades ago.

Seeing the frail finances of our proposal and recognizing the major contribution of Medicare subsidies to it, we added some features to N-HSA, to make it viable. They are explained in the following section, and make the main reason it is not possible to eliminate them in the spirit of compromise. Taken alone, some of the proposals may help. But unless the Medicare deficit is addressed in some way, the main problems will remain threatening.

Accordingly, the plan was revised to include an optional substitution of catastrophic health insurance for Obamacare, and a first and last year of life redistribution of costs to working generations. That somewhat left poor people out of the equation, so it was proposed to fund indigent people as individuals rather than through linking specific programs to them.

Nevertheless, planning such a project is worthwhile. It turns up several issues which will surely arise, even if we don't know when. That's particularly true with children, where a workable and controllable plan is offered. To the best of my knowledge, this is the first achievable proposal to be offered for children. It may well require modification, but I consider it to be a major advance just to appreciate how difficult the funding problem has always been, and how underestimated. Like everything else, it is linked to Medicare but not exclusively.

Half-way to Lifetime Health Savings Accounts

One secret of Classical Health Savings Accounts lies in recognizing that any one approach is inadequate; at least two approaches are needed. Catastrophic health insurance spreads big risks (mainly hospitalizations), while tax-free accounts promote more frugal spending for small ones (mainly ambulatory care). Combined in an HSA, they do what neither does alone, by covering overlaps. Now I contend, six principles in combination can create even greater savings, when separately they might create more confusion.

1. **Redesign Insurance.** Health insurance has traditionally been upside down. Starting with "first dollar" coverage, really sick people feared bankruptcy when medical costs outran policy limits for the last dollar. Obviously it would be better to insure big catastrophes first, skipping small ones if funds run out. If we must have mandatory health insurance, the thought ran, let it be the high-deductible catastrophic variety, with out-of-pocket limits protecting outliers. To a certain extent, the Affordable Care Act moved in that direction, possibly opening room for compromise. Deductibles should be high, but co-payments are useless, and should be eliminated. Subsidies should subsidize people, not specific programs, and should avoid taxing the program they are supporting.

2. **Indirect Transfers Between Age Groups.** Working age people largely support the health system financially but mostly don't get sick themselves, whereas sick people are mostly retired and on Medicare. That imbalance makes young people restless, while Medicare breaks the national budget with a 50% subsidy. It's largely accomplished through bond-loans from foreign countries, like China. The age-related funds transfer is desirable. But cost could be lessened by letting the worker keep health money in his HSA, earn interest, and spend it on himself when he ages. 2b. Furthermore, I propose we shift the cost of the two most expensive medical years of life to an independent fund during its period of investment. To be

specific, shift the cost of <u>the first and last years of life</u> from coverage by catastrophic health insurance and Medicare – to repaying average national cost (reported by Medicare) back to the insurers who originally paid the bills. That's familiarly known as first and last years of life re-insurance.

3. **Funds Creation.** How do we pay for this transfer? Well, in the first place, living people have somehow paid for their birth year; it will be forty more years before new ones are half-way phased in. Even terminal care costs will not level out until life expectancy stops lengthening. Revenue, on the other hand, should commence immediately. The hard part of revenue lies in "agency" failures. That is, avoid spending it in the meantime, and keeping middle-men from poaching on it. I propose individual escrow accounts are preferable to agency management by either government or private sector financial institutions. Saving for your own rainy day is much more attractive than taxing for transfers between demographic groups. The cost of passive investment in index funds is small, and long-run returns approach 11% gross, 7% net. Considering the trillions in index fund potential, these inert investments might even be considered as a substitute currency standard.

4. **Compounding.** Meanwhile it helps to recall what the Ancient Greeks knew about compound interest. Money at 7% doubles in ten years, and therefore with life expectancy now at 84, can expect to double more than eight times. 2, 4, 8, 16, 32, 64, 128, 256, (512-1024). Therefore, one dollar at birth grows to about $300 at the average time of death. By that time, life expectancy will likely grow to 94, and transforms one dollar into $500 **if** inflation is held to no more than 3%. The main hope for such price stability lies, not so much with the Federal Reserve, as in medical science reducing the burden of disease and increasing the productivity of the delivery system. I feel confident last-year costs can be covered, either by patient contribution or by government subsidy, **if** – transition costs are absorbed over a decade or so, **if** the Federal Reserve can successfully hold inflation below 3%, and **if** medical science can cure one or two major diseases in the next fifty years. Otherwise, this could be a proposal for generating tons of new revenue, but falls short of paying for all the healthcare affected. Even covering 10% would produce staggering sums, however.

Let me remind you, those extrapolations are for only one dollar invested. More specifically, the goal of the proposal is to pay for the last year of life by some variant of one-time investing of $150 at birth, possibly as much as $50 per year. This should be enough to relieve the debt pressure on Medicare, and to reduce the cost of catastrophic care for the rest of the population considerably.

5. **Adding a Generation to the Family.** For the cost of children, we propose increasing the $150 to $200 (potentially, $25 a year) and transferring the resulting surplus, **from** the grandparent's bequest **to** the Health Savings Account of no more than one grandchild at birth, thereby adding 21 years of compounding, broadening the scope to the first 21 years of life, and further reducing the premiums of catastrophic coverage for the rest of the population. Child-care costs are far more significant than they sound, because all health care plans have faltered on them. It is nearly impossible to prefund the day you are born, particularly when the responsible parents are young and financially insecure, facing the cost of an automobile, a house, a college education and another child. For a remarkably small dollar cost, compound interest can transform the social environment, and therefore I advocate the small additional cost of extending the first year of life to the first twenty-one of them.

6. **Tax Equity.** Additional required regulations are more or less self-evident, but the most important one would be to permit paying for catastrophic insurance premiums by the Health Savings Account itself, thereby creating tax exemption equivalent to employer-based insurance.

The alternative for tax equity is much more drastic – of reducing corporate tax rates, sufficient to compensate companies for losing their existing tax preference. For years, reformers have advocated tax equalization by eliminating the tax deduction for employees. It hasn't been successful, so now we advocate: equalization first, reduction later. If that is blocked, there is no choice but to lower corporate taxes, the source of the problem.

N-HSA, Bare Bones (2015 Version)

E xplanations and arguments, later. Here's the skinny on N-HSA, the plan I believe is ready to put before Congress.

CATASTROPHIC HEALTH INSURANCE

1. Everybody is assumed to have a Classical Health Savings Account. If it isn't funded, it only exists in theory.

2. Everyone who has an HSA is now required to have high-deductible catastrophic healthcare insurance coverage. This should be changed to optional coverage, which becomes mandatory if the HSA is funded in its non-escrow partition.

3. Money deposited in the non-escrowed partition may be used to pay the premium of high-deductible catastrophic insurance, making the premium as effectively tax exempt as if an employer purchased it.

4. If employer-purchased health insurance loses its tax exemption, this feature may be re-examined.

MEDICARE BUYOUT

(1. Everybody is assumed to have a Classical Health Savings Account. If it isn't funded, it is inactive.)

5. A newborn child is funded $50/yr privately, or at public expense if indigent. Payroll deductions are then added.

6. The money is passively invested in an escrowed portion of the child's HSA as a total domestic stockmarket index fund, becoming available for a Medicare buy-out at age 66 (together with accumulated payroll deductions), with the alternative of conversion into an IRA after payment of taxes. Assumed gross income rate: 11%; assumed net of inflation and transaction costs: 6.5%. Average duration: 66 years.

7. Assumed Medicare buyout price: $ 48,336 plus payroll deductions, of indeterminate amount, probably $24,000. Assumed public and private net cost: zero or near-zero (readjust #5. appropriately)..

FIRST AND LAST YEAR OF LIFE REIMBURSEMENT

8. A second escrow fund within the individual's HSA is designated to generate the funds to repay the original payer of the first and last years of life cost, using the average Medicare cost basis, thereby lowering the first-payer premiums and/or buy-out costs.

9. This has little net cost effect at first, but tends to spread the cost away from poorly financed age groups without matching increase for the working age group.

10. Estimated cost: $20/yr.

INFANTS AND CHILDREN

11. Everyone is assumed to have or is assigned one grandparent, and one grandchild. Mis-matches are pooled, or reassigned on request.

12. Grandparents are expected to bequeath the left-overs in their HSA to their grandchild's HSA, up to the limit of one child's average cost for the first 21 years of that child's life. This transfer is deemed to occur at simultaneous birth and death, and appropriate inter-fund loans or transfers are made to accomplish this.

13. This bequest does not take place to the generation who have already achieved age 21. Grandparent contributions in the first generation are pro-rated as of age 50.

14. The bequest is invested in an escrowed portion of the child's HSA as a total domestic stockmarket index fund, and transferred to his grandchild's HSA at birth for the purpose of funding. Assumed gross interest rate: 11%; assumed net of inflation and transaction costs: 6.5%. Average duration: 110 years.

INDIGENTS AND OTHER SPECIAL CASES

15. One of the great disappointments of the Obama plan is that it made health insurance mandatory, but left thirty million uninsured. It may well be true that prison inmates and mentally retarded are so different from each other, they would be better served with specialized programs than a one-size fits all.

16. Furthermore, most poor people are only poor for a portion of their lives, rising or falling with circumstances.

17. And finally treating poor people as an underclass with an attached funding source makes it impossible to have more than one program

serve them. Therefore, it seems much better to have a separate agency which addresses their poverty based on their own demonstrated preferences, than to pick winners and losers among agencies to help them.

New HSA: One Potential Solution, Several Unsolved Issues. (2014 Version)

Could a health plan stand alone, without including working-age (21-66) participation? The answer is probably negative, because the demographics are: age 21-66 supplies nearly all the money for the rest to use, when they have sickness expenses of their own to worry about. Under present circumstances, the non-working subgroup could not include subsidized costs without coordinating with Obamacare, which might now contain as much as half of healthcare costs. And as the Obamacare program evidently did, we came to recognize the thirty million uninsured have such unique needs, they are probably unsuitable for any "one size fits all" solution. Probably only a demonstration project could finally establish a final answer, but even that would take decades. Politicians are not likely to commit such huge resources without more likelihood of success.

Since these conclusions could have been reached without much study, it seems a pity they were not given more consideration before implying universal coverage would be an outcome of the Affordable Care Act. For one thing, the numbers are too large. There are about thirty million Americans who are unsuitable for anything but a subsidized program, if you only include the mentally and physically handicapped, prisoners in custody, and illegal immigrants. Since there is already an imbalance between the working well and the non-working sick, thirty million extra are just going to unbalance things more. The finances of Medicare are perhaps even more precarious than for the employed population, but there is too much public goodwill for Medicare to permit much experimentation. Decades of concealing these deficits are now returning to haunt the prospect of fixing them by any imaginable cross-subsidy.

Nevertheless, this book is a product of examining each step of the American health financing system. It may have missed some things, but it tried to be systematic. Although the attempt was made to cobble together a program for everybody omitted from the Affordable Care Act, we eventually gave up the effort as unachievable. Students of health economics may find our reasoning to be of some interest, so the essential remnants are printed in this chapter.

But one idea did emerge from this effort, which is put to work in the final synthesis in the last chapter. If it is workable, it might unravel the knotted mess of the rest of the system. **Financing the health costs of children** blocks any one-size-fits all system, pretty stubbornly, and to a greater degree than most of us realized. Some students solve the problem by dismissing its costs as trivial. They are not. Health care costs up to the 21st birthday are said by CMS to be 8% of the total lifetime costs. Since prefunding is impossible, and the legally responsible parents have precarious expenses themselves as a group, attempts are made to create family insurance plans. But since one of the two breadwinners is often impaired by the process, half of the revenue source may abruptly appear or disappear. There is a trend toward small families, but respectful provision must be made for big ones, too. With unstable family structures getting more common, and essential rights and freedoms involved, no one is really proud of the present finance designs. When you potentially start with a $27,000 deficit for every new entrant into the employment pool, there isn't much room for innovation. Nevertheless, we developed a proposal for dealing with this problem. It's at least good enough to display in public as something which will work financially, if the public can tolerate it within its social structure. I anxiously await public commentary.

In summary, it welcomes living, breathing grandparents back into the family structure. The great difference in generational ages is employed as a source of extra years for compound interest to work. The cost is presently evenly balanced between generations: one grandchild per grandparent. Because of the long period of compounding, the overall cost is less than $100 per child, not counting any net revenue from present funding sources. It thus seems fairly safe to assume it becomes self-supporting in the very long run. Even the transition costs seem containable to the age group 40-66 at about $600 total per person over three years. It would be a godsend and a bargain, if it can withstand criticism. And by lightening the family's load at a crucial moment, it might make feasible a really radical readjustment of healthcare finance. That one can be found in the very last section of the book. It's a composite of ideas, all of which are enlarged upon in different sections of the book. And even I did not anticipate where it would come out.

Proposal for Health Savings Accounts, Extended (N-HSA, 2015 Version)

On June 26, 2015, the United States Supreme Court announced its decision upholding the *status quo* of the Affordable Care Act. As Justice Jackson once put it, "We are not final because we are infallible, we are infallible only because we are final."

It would thus appear that some or all of Obamacare will continue at least until the next presidential election. For now, the Affordable Care Act is the Law, and so my immediate reaction was to propose a health care program to take care of everything else, leaving a deliberate gap from 21 to 66 untouched for whatever might be coming from the Administration, because it seems so unpredictable. What that leaves is childhood care and Medicare, plus thirty million special cases, like prison inmates, illegal immigrants, and disabled. A good case can be made that these groups differ so much, it would be better to employ five special-purpose programs rather than some one-size-fits -all approach. However, they do share some common features, and could be better integrated. For the most part, the government is their ultimate source of revenue. They are all limited in their freedom, so more supervision of the care they deliver is required. And, especially for children and prisoners, they will eventually be entitled to some of their money back at a later time. In some ways, the government acts like their trust officer.

So a Health Savings Account might well be generally suitable, since they all might need a trust officer and a guardian angel resembling a

Judge of the Orphans Court. In all the cases, there could arise special needs in their management for an accountant, a doctor, and a Judge. Foreseeing a triumvirate for supervision, and a HSA for storing the funds, the issue then arises whether it is superior to have a federal system or a more local one. Let's forget the Civil War; the federal approach confers uniformity, the state approach confers more flexibility for local control. In turn, the federal approach provides an escape hatch from local preferences. Obviously, federal prisoners will have federal supervision, and state prisoners will have state supervision, although it is questionable whether the source of the funds has much to do with the best form of supervision. Money talks, however, so this issue is probably not debatable. Nor is the issue of co-mingling of funds; the answer is a loud No. In fact, turf issues probably lead to the same response in most of these programs. In the cases of prisoners, the government must supply all the medical care, not just part of it, so voluntary Catastrophic insurance is unsuitable. All in all, you would have to ask what problem we solve with all this quarrel; ultimately you must answer for whether this new supervision is or is not superior to existing ones.

That leaves a Health Savings Account as a vehicle for funds, adding some income and possibly reducing some costs. To some extent, the HSA relies on individual responsibility, and all these people potentially have some loss of individual responsibility. Just as some Orphans Courts seem to be run by angels, others are a sickening mass of corruption, and there is no reason why this would be much different. The situation may possibly call for a blue-ribbon panel of experts to review and recommend, but scarcely calls for action to restructure everything. And it is doubtful whether the similarities of these different groups of people are greater than their differences. All these ideas have some merit, but seem more appropriate to individual adjustment, than to nationwide debate.

That is, the practical residual is addressing the healthcare of **children**, and the **elderly**. It seems – to some people – too soon to propose privatizing Medicare, since it has not sufficiently completed the process of shifting most illness costs from employer-based to itself, and has not even begun the process of shifting healthcare costs to retirement costs. Both shifts will probably occur in the next fifty years, but right now, the future of program planning is too unstable to build on. Its core problem is inability to afford the 50% government subsidy, and yet there is continuing sentiment to extend that subsidy to everybody with a "single payer" system. Fighting a battle of perceptions like that is too daunting to attempt. So what does that leave? Children.

Once you narrow the focus, you can easily see why financing the care of children has been avoided. No one has seen any way to pre-pay a newborn's health care expenses, which are reported to be 3% of the total, for the first year of life. You might as well make that 8%, and include all children up to the age of 21. The most immediate legal responsibility falls on parents who are themselves only marginally self-sufficient, many of them either unmarried or in unstable relationships. The only hopeful feature of their finances lies in the potential addition of 21 years of compound interest, if funds can somehow be transferred to use that.

I propose we overfund Medicare just a little, compound the inheritance for (on average) 83 years, and transfer it (greatly enlarged) to a grandchild's HSA at birth. Adding the two, the transfer would have 104 years to compound, and thus would require only minute amounts of seed money. My calculator reports an investment of $42 at the start will result in growth to $27,559 in 104 years. That would assume an interest rate of 6.5%, tax-free, net of 3% inflation. The revenue wouldn't look like that for 83 years, because existing grandparents are of all ages, ranging from 40 to 100, and each one would be expected to contribute catch-up revenue from birth to present age, and could stop contributing with the birth of a great-grandchild. But let's not get down into the weeds of smoothing out the payroll contributions to make the transition payments appear smaller; payroll deductions already do some of that. There's a long transition period, but the ultimate cost comes down to $42 per person per lifetime before you fudge the numbers. Meanwhile, a major problem which has defied planners for a century gets solved, and reduces the insurance costs of everyone else who was invisibly subsidizing the system. You might even increase the birthrate, which some would applaud but others would deplore.

That results in no small effort, however, because extreme versions of our focus programs require a transfer of at least 68% of healthcare costs from people who are not seriously sick, to the places where costs more naturally concentrate. The longer we wait, the worse the problem could become because of demographics. That is the case for every broad-based plan ever proposed, but this is the first one to concentrate on nothing else, because we are blocked from diluting sickness costs with the costs of well people. Since we cannot easily force well people to agree to funds transfer, we merely relieve them of the need to pay the costs, and expect they will take advantage of the opportunity. Similarly, we cannot force sick people to make use of the program, so we must rely on their recognizing the advantages.

First Year and Last Year of Life Coverage. We start with the simplest case. Everybody gets born, everyone dies; there are no exceptions. Furthermore, these two years are the most expensive ones, and are likely to remain so. Medical advances of the future may raise the costs of terminal care, but even that is uncertain, and costs may go down. It is likely to remain true that just about everybody who dies, dies at the expense of Medicare, so we start with firm data, readily available. To simplify boundary disputes, using the calendar dates of the first year and the last year eliminates that particular fuzziness. Furthermore, obstetrics and terminal care contain elements found in no other age groups, concentrating the scientific issues. When I first presented the idea to a medical audience, one wit rose to the microphone and recalled a town in Pennsylvania that passed a law stating: "Every fireplug in the town must be painted white, ten days before a fire." He was of course quizzing me how you knew when the last year of life began. The answer is, you wait until the person dies and count backward, and you get the cost data from Medicare. Since everyone knows how imprecise hospital prices may be, it is probably sufficient to reimburse average terminal care costs for the year and the region. If the patient retains Medicare coverage, a simple funds transfer to Medicare simplifies both administration and coverage disputes.

The big problem is the long transition, unless Medicare and the Administration should agree to prime the pump. Therefore, the program must remain voluntary, and may even have waiting lists at times, depending on its popularity. Certain tricks known to financial managers may help to shorten the transition to self-sufficiency. For example, CSS reports that the first year of life absorbs 3% of healthcare costs, and the last year about 6%. That is, $10,000 should be more than ample for the first year and $20,000 for the last year of life. That's assuming a lifetime medical cost of $350,000, the best estimate available. By externally supplementing the first deposits, the surplus after ten years can be applied to accelerating the funding of the last year. But even doing that could take twenty-five years to complete the process. Funds could be borrowed with a bond issue, of course, but eventually that would raise costs and prolong the transition. "Sweet spots" can be found, but at the best, the transition is a long one, certainly spanning several turnovers of political power. Nevertheless, at the end of it, these pivotal medical coverages would acquire a major funding source, and other programs could experience a major reduction, up to 9%, in cost duplication.

In this, as in other parts of the book, we round off investment returns to 7% when we really expect only 6.5%. Using the old adage that money doubles in ten years at 7%, the reader can verify approximate accuracy by doing the sums in his head as he reads.

The Rest of Childhood, Seniority, and Permanent Unemployability. So that was the first **Proposal 21:**, to which the second one is a natural extension. All children are dependents of their parents, and the heavy costs of obstetrics (magnified by the unusual concentration of malpractice claims) make it impossible to devise pre-funding schemes. Young parents are often strapped for funds, so the lack of pre-funding is a growing problem in a Society uncertain of its family structures. Therefore, we have devised the **grandparent roll-over**. Tort reform would improve but not eliminate this work-around. Therefore children are lumped with senior citizen costs, and hence to a gradual buy-out of Medicare.

The permanently unemployable are included by using surplus funds from the other two, mainly because there is no way to establish eligibility except by starting a program and seeing what it costs if you monitor it. Those may not seem like adequate reasons to lump them together, but it will be seen the details feel congenial, to do so. That is always a good sign in new proposals.

Multiple Programs in Multiple Years. The transition problem is always vexing in a new program, but reaches some sort of new limit when the ambition is to work toward uniformity and maximum patient control, across the entire nation; fragmentation always sounds easier. The temptation is always there to issue orders and threaten to use force, but it must be resisted. Furthermore, enormous cost savings are readily available if programs are multi-year, and cost is a paramount issue, here. It's hard to beat compound interest, the longer the better.

To explain the reasoning of the grandpa transfer mainly requires the observation that grandparents are comparatively new re-entrants to the average family. It's simple (one grandchild's worth of costs, per person), it uses surplus cash after a grandpa has no further use for it, and it comes at an optimum time on the compound interest curve. It greatly stretches the lifetime for compounding, but it is also readily suited for a limitation on perpetuity. It even follows established family patterns, although families are under considerable stress, these days. True, it jumps over a new barrier for the first time, but it doubles the duration of compounding, skips over the issue of leaving a dark hole around the Obamacare age group, skips over the contentious issues of pre-funding obstetrics, simplifying a host of unnecessary red tape obstacles. And it reduces costs by half.

No Employer Involvement, No Obamacare Contributions. At first, it seems like a relief not to have to deal with the two thorniest issues of the past, but in fact it doesn't quite do that. If the patient has duplicate coverage, there must be cordial negotiations to see which coverage should be dropped. And while significant savings can be readily demonstrated, there will be some residual revenues which have to be transferred along with the patient, or the new program will starve. The complicated systems we have evolved to facilitate cost-shifting will probably invalidate old statistics, and perhaps some old ideas. Transferring six percent of the gross domestic product is by definition a tedious, difficult task, even if you reduce it to four percent in the process. Everyone is hesitant to name the individuals who will lose their jobs, or their pensions, or their seniority, if the program shifts significantly. But if the savings aren't significant, what good are they?

New Health Savings Accounts (N-HSA)

O n June 26, 2015, the United States Supreme Court handed down its opinion on *King v. Burwell*, essentially leaving the Affordable Care Act unchanged. Much will be written about this controversial opinion, but little of it would have to do with Health Savings Accounts.

> If anyone is interested in my opinion about the contested language in the law, it is derived from reading Jacob S. Hacker's book about the passage of the Clinton Health Plan, called *The Road to Nowhere*. The plan as described by Hacker, was to plant deliberately conflicting proposals in the House and Senate bills, so the real proposal could remain concealed until the House-Senate conference committee meeting, where the versions meant to survive could be identified. The final result could thus be released when the press was absent, preferably on the eve of a holiday.

> It didn't happen in the case of Hillary Clinton's plan (which was never fully released), while in the case of President Obama's Plan, it was suspended in mid-operation by the death of Senator Kennedy. But the Senate version had been passed by a friendly Senate, so the House was forced to vote on an identical bill, to *avoid* returning to a conference committee convened by a newly hostile Senate. This version of the story fits the known facts pretty well, and is reinforced by Hacker's subsequent membership on the Obama election team. Unfortunately, the Supreme Court's later decision constitutes an endorsement of a parliamentary maneuver which ought to be forbidden. Let's now break off this conjecture, and return to Health Savings Accounts.

My original intent in 2014 was to offer **Lifetime Health Savings Accounts (L-HSA)** in such a way the two programs (ACA and HSA) could be negotiated into a compromise that both could live with. In time, they would eventually evolve into hybrids that both would be proud of, or else lead the voters to state a clear preference for either one to be exclusive, after they had a taste of both. Offhand, I could see no value for either one to be declared mandatory, if that would still leave 30 or so million people uninsured. "Mandatory" did not seem like a helpful word to use, and often it seemed harmful to someone. In applying a computer search engine to the Affordable Care Act, I was unable to find a single use of the word "mandatory". Looking back on it, its premise was flawed but its intent was felt to be benign, so perhaps face-saving boilerplate was called for.

The central feature of the Savings Account has always revolved around the fact that youthful health care is usually cheap, while health care for the elderly is expensive. Many decades of tax-free compound interest at 6.5% would thus have been allowed to build up in some sort of escrow under both plans, until the age when healthcare really gets expensive. At that point it would not matter which program it was assisting, and both sides would stop looking for a victory. By that time, I wouldn't be surprised if the deficits of the Medicare program had become so fearsome, and the debts of the program become so threatening, that both sides would be willing to consider modifications of Medicare. If not, subscribers to a buy-out had built up a six-figure retirement fund.

Medicare is already more than 50% subsidized by taxes and foreign borrowing, but the public scarcely knows it. I believe it is just a matter of time before the public realizes where it is going, but right now they see Medicare as getting a dollar's worth of healthcare for 50 cents, if they think about it at all. I suspect it would take a full year or more of intense Congressional work to fill in the action details of a lifetime or lifecycle system, and maybe longer than that to re-direct public opinion. The proposal is voluntary, no politician dares to force it down anyone's throat. And the proposed incremental steps would also be voluntary. The investments would be in personal accounts, so no one could divert them for aircraft carriers. And the accounts would be lucrative, so no one needs to be afraid of their solvency.

Because compound interest on savings from the working years tends to rise after about age 45, a long period of Health Savings Accounts generates much more money than from a string of disconnected single years. Like the difference between term insurance and whole-life insurance, you can't judge the improved investment of L-HSA by multiplying one C-HSA times your life expectancy, so it is a subtlety that two continuous programs would generate more funds than two separated ones.

Meanwhile, we have **Classical Health Savings Accounts (C-HSA)** which already have more than 15 million satisfied subscribers, steadily growing in number. Most of the Obamacare subscribers wouldn't want HSAs, and most of the HSA subscribers wouldn't consider the ACA plan, so total insured would increase. HSAs are described in the first chapter of this book, and in 35 years only about four or five improvements have come along, awaiting Congressional approval, but bipartisan passage of them would calm the waters considerably. They need a tax deduction for the Catastrophic health insurance premiums, to make their owners just like everyone else. The easiest way to accomplish this is to extend permission for the Accounts themselves (which are tax exempt) to purchase the catastrophic insurance which is required. Catastrophic health insurance is itself tangled in Obamacare regulations, which need to be revised, to deserve Presidential signature from any President. The annual deposit limits now need to be liberalized, and restated as total lifetime limits to account for the varying ages of new subscribers.

And new regulations need to accommodate the new phenomenon of *passive* investing, which is deservedly sweeping the nation, providing much lower transaction costs and higher average returns, which might be made still higher. Although HSAs are mostly self-administered, new investment managers are a little afraid of them, and well established firms do not yet seem to recognize their enormous long-term potential. For these reasons, many early investors have been "savvy financial people", an image I am very anxious to see change to "ordinary folks", without resulting in "high fees for rubes".

To return to the Supreme Court's *King* decision, the only version of HSA which is ready to go is the Classical one, which would still be improved by a few amendments, if the President is of a mind to cooperate. His own plan seems more or less in suspense, waiting for Big Business to emerge from its policy huddle, after two years of delay. Many tradeoffs and compromises can be envisioned for that coordination, of by far the biggest eligible group of subscribers. It is my commentary that employers' gift of health insurance in 1945 has long since been compensated for, by a corresponding drop in wages.

So nothing but a tax exemption is left. The amount of money involved is so huge, it requires other issues be brought into the discussion to avoid a stock market panic. It particularly needs to be emphasized that a loophole based on the corporate income tax rate is not at all – not at all – the same as an increase or decrease of corporate income at that rate. Getting a free lollipop at a 60% discount, does not affect your company's income by 60%.

Nevertheless, the existence of fringe benefit tax dodges does create pressure to retain the high corporate taxes, and those taxes need to be reduced to keep our corporations from fleeing to tax havens abroad. My suggestion is to lower the corporate income tax in parallel with a comparable reduction of the employer tax dodge, a maneuver so delicate it ought to be overseen by the Federal Reserve, acting under a Congressional time limit. Such a proposal is so newsworthy it might well suck the air out of the room for Health Savings Accounts, and Obamacare, too. Everyone involved has an incentive to be cautious and reasonable, a difficult thing to be, during an election year. However with prudence, breaking the logjam on the migration of American corporations to foreign locations could be the thing which suddenly gets everyone's attention.

New Health Savings Accounts (N-HSA)

Because it increasingly seems so unlikely a notoriously stubborn President would ditch his health plan at this late date, I turned my attention to seeing what could be done with using Health Savings Accounts for what's left. Obamacare is likely to be subject to twists and turns until after the November 2016 elections, and this administration has a history of preferring to operate out of sight. Therefore, my revised plan was to avoid the subject as much as possible, except for one thing. The savings in a portion of the Account would continue to accumulate as a tax-exempt investment account, available for extra medical expenses until age 66, when it turns into a retirement account. That is, a N-HSA account could exist untouched for as many as 45 years (21-66) without a catastrophic backup insurance, or else if agreeable, with a catastrophic policy coordinated with an Obamacare policy. The purpose of this part of the structure was to provide a haven for long-term buildup of funds, with as few financial drains on it as possible, while it stays out of the way. On the other hand, money seems no good if you can't spend it, so it needs some contingency exits.

It is possible to summarize a great deal of thinking by stating that it mostly can't be done. The evolution in healthcare has not reached the point where people aged 21 to 66 could save enough to support the rest of the population, while taking care of their own health. In fifteen years that might become possible, but not yet. Even then, an additional thirty million people who are unemployable (prisoners in custody, disabled people, and illegal immigrants) would probably topple the system without some major reductions in the cost of chronic diseases (diabetes, Alzheimers, arthritis, emphysema, kidney failure) which might well take another fifty years. So we temporarily set this attractive idea aside.

Except for one thing, paying for children under 21. The system devised was to overfund Medicare slightly, gather investment income for a combined 104 years, and transfer the result to a grandchild or pool of grandchildren to pay for 21 years of healthcare. The grandparent transfers the money at death after 83 years of compounding, but the child receives a lump sum at birth and erodes it to near zero by the 21st birthday. This is how 104 years are available to the next generation to grow a contribution of $42 to $27,000, while staying within the limits of the Law of Perpetuities. To do this requires passive investing of a total-stock index averaging 6.5% net of 3% inflation. According to records by students of the subject, the total stock market has averaged 11% returns for a century, in spite of wars and depressions. Right now, the main obstacle to achieving this is the community of middle-men in the financial world. It the problem continues to be a stubborn one, I advise taking delivery on the stock index security, putting it in a safe deposit box, and opening it decades later.

One issue comes up, that this system could produce unlimited amounts of inflated money by escalating the initial single payment. But it cannot do so if the account balance starts from, or must go to, zero. If loopholes are discovered, additional points of zero balance could be imposed.

Medicare Backup Insurance. In the original planning of Health Savings Accounts, it never seemed likely we would lack places to spend money ear-marked for healthcare. However, 45 years really is a long time to have your money locked out of reach. The other side of this coin is the spectacular result of long-term passive investing. Just to throw in a couple of examples, the investment of $1000 at age 21 would result in a fund of $16,000 at age 66, and an investment of $1000 a year, every year from 21-66, would accumulate a fund of $246,375 at age 66, quite a nice retirement fund. And if you were lucky enough to live frugally, from 66 to 83 the $16,000 would grow to $43,800, and the $246,000 would grow to $680,165. If you grow uneasy about Medicare solvency, these sums would be nice to have in the bank. In effect, they could serve the function of catastrophic self-insurance, without the insurance.

As a matter of fact, it would be nice to include a provision that the Health Savings Account could dispense with the expense of catastrophic insurance when it grows to a point equaling it. It would dramatize the subtle transformation, from an account for drugstore expenses, into a serious investment tool. That won't happen soon, and it won't happen to everyone, but it is a realistic goal.

Healthcare for Children. Now, that leads into an entirely different direction. One of the perpetual headaches of designing health care finance, is the fact that newborn babies are expensive. Part of that is due to inordinate malpractice costs for obstetrics, partly it is due to expensive care being devoted to premature babies and Caesarian sections. But mainly it is due to the parents being young people without much savings. It's pretty hard to design a pre-funded health care plan for an individual who starts the second year of life with a $10,000 debt.

His parents barely climb out of a financial hole before the child himself is ready to have children. As we have seen in earlier paragraphs, some frugal grandparents end up with more healthcare money than they can spend on their own health. American mothers average 2.1 babies apiece, and with a little fumbling it can be seen, that figure averages one grandchild per grandparent. If aggregate health care for children 0-21 averages $29,000, Grandpa could give a child a very nice start on life by rolling over his surplus at age 83 to a grandchild at birth – if the laws permit such a thing, particularly if no family connection exists. (We'll have to leave unorthodox family sexual preferences to the matrimonial lawyers to sort out.)

With ingenuity, an additional 21 years can be added to the period of compound interest, and we've already shown what a difference that can make in an 83 (or maybe 93) year lifespan. In case you missed the point, when Grandpa relieves the cost of healthcare for a grandchild, the benefit is indirectly felt by the child's parents, although that isn't invariably true. Right now, the cost of a child's healthcare is the responsibility of the parent, so it's relatively fair.

Payroll Deductions and Premiums for Medicare. With 300 million citizens, a lot of exceptional cases can arise, and the foregoing probably doesn't contain enough incentives to start a stampede for N-HSA. Accordingly, let's consider forgiving the Medicare payroll deduction, in whole or in part, as a legitimate spending outlet. And if that isn't enough, consider waiving Medicare premiums. Both of these are legitimate health costs, so no one is violating the purpose of a tax deduction for Health Savings Accounts. Each one of them covers about a quarter of Medicare costs, so the funds are ample. (The present average costs of Medicare are about $180,000 per lifetime).

And finally, there's your Social Security contribution. SS isn't a medical cost, but it's a retirement cost, and that's what N-HSA could turn into. Reducing any or all of these expenses will free up a comparable amount of spendable income. If all else fails, consider abating your income tax. Income tax isn't a health expense, but it is often the largest item in a retiree budget. Reducing income tax could displace other funds designated for health costs, and hence indirectly could sometimes be considered a health cost, itself. There are plenty of ways to create savings with the government, and all you probably really need is their permission to do it.

To repeat, the purpose of all this is to find a way to subsidize the health expenses of children, which in my view is the unsuspected stumbling block for all self-funded lifetime proposals. Even the tax-evasive employer-based system gets into a tangle over it.

Subsidies for the Poor. We must conclude by mentioning poor people. It's of course true you have to start with some money to earn income from it. What are you going to offer poor folks, when the country is already deeply in debt? Well, it's practically impossible to say what Obamacare is going to do for them, although it will surely do what it can. The possibility of double-subsidies is still present, when the situation is as unstable as it is, and the economy is as fragile as it is. So this proposal prefers to delay the subsidy discussion until Obamacare is also on the table.

To facilitate that discussion, this plan has been forced to organize the subsidy money for poor folks to come out of the age group 21-66, who are effectively the only real creators of wealth in the whole system. That coincides with Obamacare, and cannot be effectively discussed without including it. However, once it is coordinated, the subsidy to poor people could be quite substantial as a result of being placed at the far end of the compound interest curve, and given enough years to work in an escrow account. If if came to a showdown, the subscriber could take delivery on an index fund certificate, and put it in a bank lockbox until it was needed. I propose separating subsidies from all healthcare, and funding them independently. Independent of the intermediaries of their grants, that is.

To summarize, we start with a regular Health Savings Account with obstructions removed. In return for allowing the HSA to remain in the background, gathering interest, the HSA effectively assists Medicare. Assisting Medicare could mean helping in a Medicare buy-out, or it could be used to help Social Security. Or it could recirculate through Grandpa, to help the coming generation. An option for Grandpa to make the choice would simplify administration, but possibly unbalance something else.

Coordinating New HSA with The Affordable Care Act.

Starting with N-HSA We have just described the general outline of New Health Savings Accounts (N-HSA). Essentially, it consists of individual HSA funds for children, connected to Medicare by permitting the funds to sit in escrow from age 21 to age 66. However, the amount which can be accumulated during childhood is small, and the task it is asked to perform is large. Because children are so lacking in income, they can't be expected to accumulate much, even though their grandparents may have helped out. Consequently, that small amount multiplied by compounded income for 45 years, will probably only pay for one designated segment of the Medicare program, and it is unlikely it would be able to pay off much of Medicare's accumulated debt.

So, although it can be shown to be workable, it would look like a long run for a short slide, to an economically illiterate family. Meanwhile, its political enemies would likely describe it as meddling with Medicare, and its chances of achieving the necessary enablements would shrink. However, the grand discovery is, the Health Savings Account idea resembles how President John Adams once described his native Boston – Every goose is a swan. Every problem we encounter, that is, seems to suggest an unexpected new improvement. Let's explain the three accompanying graphs.

Three Graphs. The top graph shows the situation, without either a bridge around, or participation in, the Affordable Care Act. The HSA escrow comes to a halt for 45 years, and then resumes with Medicare. There are two savings accounts, but each starts at zero and lasts two decades. One is an escrow account, unspendable until age 66.

The middle graph imagines the situation with a dormant escrow gathering interest during the 45 years. Notice the thickened blue escrow.

The bottom graph is a cutout enlargement of the transfer point for grandpa's gift, showing how easy it would be to adjust the escrow transfer from zero to $29,000. The difference between the extremes added to the escrow is the difference between solvency and riches. To imagine a small deposit spiralling out of control is probably a little fanciful, but for those who worry, here is a ready solution.

Adding Obamacare. If we achieve political consensus, and thereby add the subscribers from age 21 to 66 (the only age group which reliably produces real new wealth), the arithmetic suddenly transforms. The complete system from cradle to grave generates enormous surpluses. After studying this paradox for some time, I came to realize that what distinguished it from Lifetime Health Savings Accounts (L-HSA) was the two, eventually three, breaks between programs, where the escrow fund could drop to zero, without some agreement to transfer it between insurance programs. If it drops to zero, the effect of compound interest rising at its far end is chopped off, and overall returns are much reduced. The whole idea unfortunately then becomes politically precarious, and runs the risk of some small glitch somewhere unraveling it. To use our own descriptive terms, three Classical (C-HSA) funds are nice, but one Lifetime (L-HSA) is so far superior it raises grandiose questions of starting an inflationary spiral. But in a sense, the radical Right is correct. The changes to the Affordable Care Act must be drastic enough to generate public support for merging the radical plan of the left with a radical plan of the right, essentially making both of them unrecognizable. I'm no politician, but I can easily imagine the difficulties of that negotiation.

The Goose is a Swan. But I came to see that what makes it impractical is the same as what makes it so glamorous. The possibility of linking the healthcare fund to the stock market would likely be brushed aside by the explosions of a money machine – the system as originally envisioned for L-HSA generates almost any amount of money you please. That's a pretty intolerable effect of inflation heedlessly disregarding any monetary standard, even a return of a gold standard

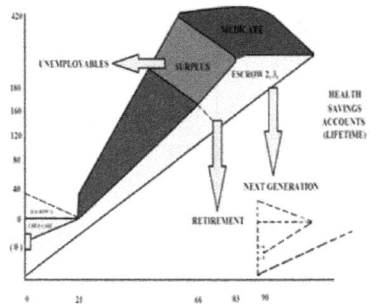

But if the HSA is more or less denominated in index funds, it essentially has a monetary standard built in, and could maintain it if someone held a meat ax in reserve. Some impregnable threat is needed to control the monster, and it is provided at the three linkage points, where the three existing insurance programs connect.

Three Meat Axes. The connection after the children's escrow fund is the most leveraged and therefore the most sensitive, since we have already demonstrated how the difference between zero transfer between two funds, and the transfer of $27,000, is the difference between marginally paying Medicare bills, and having money to burn. If some totally reliable monetary angel could be discovered and put in charge of it, the discretion about inflationary consequences could be placed in one pair of hands.

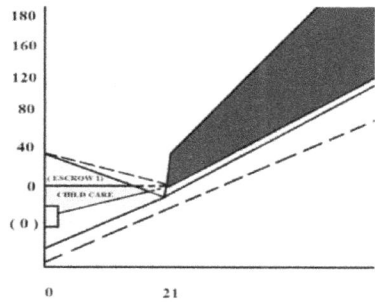

But the history of inflation has been that even Kings, Popes and Emperors have succumbed to the temptations of such power. Remember, this fund is truly generating $350,000 of new wealth per person (in a nation of 300 million inhabitants) if it operates precisely as hoped, so it starts with some latitude. There are several Presidents of the nations of the world, who might fairly be suspected of raiding their own currency right at this moment, however. Wisdom suggests more caution is necessary. For example, Congress could permit a discretionary band within which the Executive branch could operate, perhaps in consultation with the Federal Reserve. That might permit Congress to create some very difficult hurdle for the process to jump, for widening the limits of the band, such as a Constitutional Amendment.

There's an End in Sight. And also remember, my colleagues in the research department are busy looking for a cure for cancer and Alzheimer's Disease, and I feel confident they will eventually have success. Just cure diabetes, schizophrenia, or birth defects, and our problem with Health Savings Accounts would transform into how to turn them off. In the meantime, we must modulate the ups and downs of medical costs which are steadily becoming less urgent. Take warning from the recent example of the price of tetracycline, which a year or two ago was 35 cents retail for fifty capsules, and suddenly jumped to $3.50 for a single capsule. And then with a new owner, jumped to thousand of dollars. If things like that continue to happen, we might be ready for another pet scheme of mine, the limitation of health insurance coverage to covering the first year of life, and the last year of life, by eliminating most of the disease in-between. Because of the helplessness of both these population groups, and the universality of the need for their coverage, in their case alone drastic interference with market mechanisms might appear justified, to those who are injured by them. The rest of us ought to have a say in something like that. But that's another book, for another time.

We're some way from seriously having that type of problem, so let's get back to details. For this purpose, paying patients arrange themselves into only three groups, children, working folks, and Medicare recipients. Thus there exist three breakpoints between these three programs for different ages, assuming Congress authorizes transfers between them, especially from grandparent generation to grandchildren, incidentally relieving the middle generation of a lot of cost-shifting. There is now so much (necessary) cost shifting, it is nearly impossible to sort out the cost numbers. So I won't try to do it, except in a sort of general way. Rationing is a sort of a lip-service concession to the wide-spread liberal endorsement of a single payer system, endorsing but without facing the resultant deficits in every direction. Instead, we encounter the worrisome potential for generating too much money, even though that is hard to believe without endorsing galloping inflation. There is little difference between external transfers – between insurance plans, and internal transfers – within one mega-institution – except in this case one approach creates impossible deficits, and the other approach raises a realistic concern about inflation. A compromise might be devised, but it requires some sort of conciliatory response from the both sides, for even a beginning.

Meanwhile, I don't scoff at the legal issues of who is responsible for whose bills, if we destroy the family unit with exciting new social liberties. And I haven't forgotten the problem of corporate finance officers, who have run a confidence game for eighty years, making money for the stockholders by giving away health insurance to employees, as long as they can conceal what they are really doing. We've suggested in this book, we should offer business a reduction of their corporate income tax to levels comparable to individual tax levels, in return for getting them out of the health insurance business.

In a sense, it returns the favor of making a profit by giving away a service benefit, by – generating revenue for the public sector in return for reduced taxes in the private sector. I'm entirely serious about offering major corporations a one percent cut in corporate taxes for each two percent reduction in fringe benefit tax exemption, down to the point where top corporate income tax rate is equal to the average individual tax rate. That benchmark is selected because of the temptation otherwise created, to elect Subchapter C to S inter-conversions, exploiting such tax differences. International corporate flight is another serious consideration. Meanwhile, it is always possible to equalize employee tax exemption by allowing HSAs to purchase catastrophic insurance through the HSA itself, if the law would permit it.

Inflation Protection. Q. Now, wait a minute. If we permit a money machine to be built, what is to prevent it from resembling the galloping inflation which ruined the Weimar Republic? And if we devise a way to keep the United States from going down that road, how do we prevent a hundred small foreign states (Zimbabwe, for instance) from doing it deliberately in order to use their sovereign status to acquire the index funds held by Health Savings Accounts?

A. You've almost answered your own question about Zimbabwe. Even without freely floating currencies, the markets are quick to detect changes in the value of foreign currency. Zimbabwe can force its own people to accept pennies disguised as trillion-dollar bills, but everybody else avoids them, whereas bitcoins don't even have sovereign power. And as for our own domestic currency, I propose we enact a band of fluctuation in consultation with the Federal Reserve, within which the dollar can float, and beyond which the band may not be expanded without a Constitutional Amendment, again in consultation with the Federal Reserve. In two hundred years, the amendment process has only let one matter (Prohibition of alcohol) slip past, which had to be revoked after experience with it. Almost every other indiscretion has proved to crumble in spite of temptation to raid the cookie jar.

Watchdogs. Three breakpoints, one between each age group, with wildly different medical needs and financial viewpoints, need watchdogs. Since going to zero between any two of the three insurance programs could bring inflation to a halt, and since venality knows no political boundaries, I suggest each break point be governed by a different political entity, composed of a board nominated by a different branch of government, and each ratified by a different process. It may or may not be necessary for them to share the same information agency, since think tanks are very popular right now, but may not continue to be. We will need another conference in a resort hotel to work out a paper, but keep in mind that foreign powers will be anxious to infiltrate and subvert it. So maybe we need two conferences, one to review the other. After all, we are talking about 18% of the gross domestic product, and Benjamin Franklin isn't available any more.

What's the Matter With Medicare? And Single-Payer?

With great reluctance, I feel I must discuss adding the option to buy out of Medicare. I am a happy satisfied patient of that program, and for many decades was a happy, satisfied provider of care under it. Prior to 1965, I practiced medicine for 15 years before there was a Medicare program, so I have something to compare it with. The main difference I see is the tremendous backlog of untreated chronic conditions which had built up during the Great Depression of the Thirties, followed by the war years. Let me describe it; but remember, my final conclusion is "Sorry, Medicare, but we've outgrown you."

In those early days, every mouth I opened hid snaggly teeth, every other eardrum seemed to be perforated. The smelly weeping varicose ulcers of the legs were hard to take, but there were hernias and gallstones galore. And hemorrhoids, and stomach ulcers. Most eyes seemed to have cataracts growing in them, the goiters were as big as grapefruit. From the doctor's point of view, the disease burden of the population was never going to be exhausted. We scarcely realized we were dealing with a backlog, and tended to believe this was just the way poor people had to live. In fact, we cleared out that backlog in ten years, scarcely realizing it was diminishing. Meanwhile, we built up another backlog, so to speak, of a population whose disease burden had been cleared away. Re-building that healthy reserve was a sort of ghoulish reserve against some blunder we could coast through. Because, like it or not, some people will neglect their health if we stop making treatment free.

If we now have another depression or war, we could probably coast through the lack of optional medical treatment for several years, believing all the while, the cost of healthcare was decreasing. Treating the backlog is one of the costs of Medicare which never seems to get counted, and doing away with it left us with an unmeasurable reserve of artificially healthy patients. And it wasn't just minor conditions with optional treatments. When I was a visiting consultant at Philadelphia General Hospital, it was not unusual to visit the autopsy room before we went to the wards, and the residents would present several, perhaps five, bodies on the slabs. Following that, we would go upstairs to the 40-bed wards and make rounds on the patients who might well occupy the slabs on another day, because they had been too far gone when they arrived.

Present day residents have little comprehension of the devastating severity of disease we had before us, and administrators have little idea of the change this has made in costs. When we needed all this equipment we often didn't have it; nowadays the residents have a lot of equipment they seldom use. Some of this would have improved without Medicare, but Medicare certainly hurried it up. You don't hear many doctors of my generation criticizing Medicare.

Just what the patients thought of it all, is hard to judge. By the nature of things, the sick people were older than the doctors who treated them, and the doctors are now in their nineties. I get the feeling the old folks are deathly afraid Medicare will be stripped of funding in order to pay for the unaffordable Affordable Care Act. So they are ambiguous; they got a lucky break which they don't want to deny to younger people. But they seem to recognize the costs are unsupportable. They silently read the Sunday newspaper columns about the $10,000 pills for cancer. Like me, they see a two-page listing of hospital administrators making $4 million annual salaries, with the listing going down to $250 thousand per year before the newspaper runs out of space. The old folks know almost nothing about the Affordable Care Act, but they immediately recognize that such articles are written to stir up animosity to hospital costs. They don't know what to think, so they appear to have decided it is best to keep their heads low. All they seem to want is a chance to have their share of it, before it all goes away.

And they should feel the way they do. When Secretary Sibelius published the Medicare balance sheet, I was astounded to see the program is only 50% self-supporting, the rest is borrowed from the general fund. And everybody knows the general fund is largely borrowed from the Chinese, who are in financial distress themselves, right now. Books are in print accusing the government of desiring more inflation, in order to cause effective default on our sales of Treasury bonds to (i.e., borrowing from) the Chinese. Medicare recipients showed little interest in the Obamacare debate, and therefore have almost no information about it. But they grasped the essential point, all right. Medicare is delivering a dollar's worth of healthcare for fifty cents. And everyone in Congress is scared to death to bring up the subject, for fear they touch the third rail of politics.

Aside from that rather considerable political matter, there are a number of basic flaws in Medicare. Medicare has a monopoly of healthcare for the elderly. It doesn't have to be mandatory. A 50% discount below cost would quickly make almost anything at all substantially mandatory. All monopolies inhibit competition, especially in adopting innovation, and all of them ultimately thrive on shortages. The breakup of the ATT monopoly unleashed a flood of pent-up innovation in the telephone field, for a familiar illustration.

The inevitable domination of a field by an extra-large competitor is dramatically illustrated by California's present dominance of insurance design. Essentially all new designs of insurance feel they must first conform to California's regulations, and if necessary just ignore the smallest states. That's a current example of what John Dickinson was afraid of at the Constitutional Convention. He was simultaneously Governor of Pennsylvania, one of the largest states, and of Delaware, one of the smallest. He knew what he was talking about, and essentially that is why we have a Senate with two votes per state, regardless of population. This analysis ought to be known as the Dickinson Concept, because it is one of the main reasons our Constitution has survived for two hundred years, while every single other constitution has floundered. Monopolies are usually very bad things, but in a very subtle way. And yet bigness is a sign of success in a company. It's a very subtle distinction.

In the case of healthcare, we have a nationwide system of one-price-fits all, making no distinction in price between good and bad care, or whether the patient lives or dies. Obamacare recognizes this flaw and has appointed a committee to look into fixing it. Lots of luck with that, because the nation recognizes the unwisdom of letting government pick winners and losers. It probably just can't be done acceptably. State-wide uniform prices are about the best you can do with either a command-and-control system or an insurance system. Haggling in a marketplace is treated with disdain, but it's the only way anyone has devised, to reward good quality. So, a nationwide Medicare encounters this problem, and enlarging it to nationwide single payer, would make it even more troublesome. Everyone can see that Wisconsin benefits when Illinois tries to do it.

Nationwide uniformity has some advantages, such as concentrating essentially all the deaths in one program for research, although the bigdata computer approach may eliminate even that edge. What a monopoly tends to do, is enlarge one institution's scope until it finally gets so top-heavy it collapses. How many corporations can you name who are a hundred years old? The curse of bigness is so powerful that only those who have experienced it, can anticipate it. The big gorilla dominates so insidiously, the competitors forget how to compete. Everything is wonderful, until suddenly it is terrible.

And finally, the greatest problem with healthcare is its design. By insuring the cheap stuff but running out of money when you really need it, we are killing the Canary in the Coal Mine. Front-end deductible reverses that perverse priority. It corrects a system that will only work if you eliminate most disease, big and small. The advance of science is relentlessly crowding serious illness into the age group over 66, and is eventually destined to trivialize medical care in younger healthier people. Eventually we will get, or possibly have already started to get, a system so focused on the present, it fails to look to the future. Eighteen percent of the gross domestic product is being transferred from people who will have never felt a wound, to the non-working minority over 66, who will eventually have serious illness all to themselves. The people who don't have much sickness are expected to pay for the old folks, who do. It's a prescription for rebellion, and perhaps some of the present travail is already a sign of it. I'm sorry to have to tell this to my fellow subscribers to Medicare, but if you become too expensive, the kids may ditch you. I'm already older than most people on Medicare, and you will notice I'm still struggling to design an alternative to this wonderful half-price bargain. It's tough, because even cutting the cost in half will leave the impression prices were unchanged. That's because the gains and losses were hidden in the public sector, with only the gains getting some publicity.

So, the conclusion is this. If the politicians are right and Medicare is untouchable, the main danger is its reputation will entice us to extend it further, as a "Single Payer" system for everybody. At a dollar for fifty cents, even an exorbitantly expensive system seems to be a bargain. So a last-ditch warning by implication is this: Follow the doctor's advice, in Latin, of *Primum non nocere.* If you can't make things better, for pity's sake, don't make things worse.

Medicare Buy-Out

C ould Americans buy their way out of Medicare? Right now, no. In a few years, probably yes. A Medicare buy-out would have a few special complications. The transition to it might take thirty or more years, in view of the several ways it raises revenue, and the varying ages of the patients involved. For example, from the time an individual starts his first job, until the age of 66, he is sustaining payroll deductions for future Medicare coverage. Also, from the age of 66 until he dies, he has Medicare premiums deducted from his Social Security payments. Each of these compartments aggregates about a quarter of the cost of the program, and the two methods keep more or less in balance over a lifetime, eventually paying half its cost.

The other half of the Medicare program cost is supplied through general tax sources, as a subsidy, and could continue to build up indefinitely. Eventually, an undeterminable portion of the subsidy is borrowed internationally, and that debt, like a credit-card balance, draws continuous interest. The *Economist* reports it would be more advantageous for the Chinese to buy American common stock. But using that approach, they would now own a fifth of the major corporations of America, which is politically unacceptable. Therefore, they bought American Treasury bonds. Depending on maturity, these bonds will eventually come due and must then be redeemed or refinanced. This arrangement can only continue with mutual consent of the two nations, and currently the Chinese economy is shaky.

Moreover, it cannot be said the two funds will keep in balance. That's essentially true in bulk, but the actual revenue for each age cohort is largely based on its historical birth rate. Payroll deductions for the baby boom bulge have reached a peak and are about to decline to zero, whereas the Medicare premium bulge is just beginning, along with benefit payments. These repeated imbalances could prove troublesome to fund.

I wish I believed these receipts had been put into a bank vault, but in fact they were likely co-mingled for general government expenses, and spent long ago. Whether or not they are represented by accountants as paying for part of future Medicare expenses, or for current bridges and battleships, they are going to make a problem when the boomer bulge catches up with them. The formula will remain unchanged, but the proportion of payroll deducters will fall because the Millennial generation are fewer than the boomer generation, who are in turn more numerous than their parents as consumers of Medicare funds. The Treasury would certainly be concerned about any proposal to accelerate the payout to help a Medicare buyout. And even if an exchange of health funding is agreed to, the accounting problem of determining millions of balances of differing size is sure to be a headache. The balance in question is the net of 6.5%, less the rate on Treasury bonds, which could be either a positive balance or a negative one, if the bond market and the stock market do not move in parallel. The unpredictability of markets is amply illustrated at present, when trillions of freshly printed bonds do not cause inflation, even for the mundane purpose of maintaining a stable currency. Even inflation targeting does not work as desired, currently reaching 1.5% when the Federal Reserve is trying to reach 2%.

In the longer run, Medicare buy-outs by the grandchild approach would stretch available funds over a longer time span, and augment them somewhat. Longevity is increasing, but the period of working life is not. People are retiring earlier, and they are entering the workforce later in life. Progressive taxation further reduces what working people have left over to spend, and eventually will make them less willing to support the protracted vacations of their children and their parents. So extra investment income will be needed, and shifting other savings around will probably relieve some of the pressure. Even so, it appears certain some elderly people will outlive their savings, and must find a way to generate income with their leisure time. Along the same lines, we must also change the mentality of those who regard employment as a punishment to be avoided, but that is not my present topic. One small advantage of the unemployed Millennials is they are less likely to resist working longer after they do get a job.

Summary of One Scheme of Medicare Buyout. A childhood health insurance, funded through a health insurance for senior citizens. Owned by two people linked by redefining a birthday or some other strategy, all sounds like a peculiar idea. But let me persuade you to do a little math. At 7%, there are 9 doublings in a 90 year life. 2, 4, 8, 16, 32, 64, 128, 256, 512. That's rounding up on 6.5% and 85 years, which are closer to realistic estimates of future longevity and interest rate return, but no one can predict. Every dollar at birth (now redefined financially as the 21st birthday) is multiplied 512 times. The grandparent aged 40 would have to add $450 to a sinking fund, and a grandparent aged 65 would have to contribute $27,000 to pay it in advance. Eventually, when things settle down and we have added four doublings, the contribution would be $42 a person, so considerable juggling would be useful for a few years to smooth it out fairly.

Let's aim for $200 a year for five or ten years for everybody over age 40, or something of that nature. To pay for Medicare coverage, that's amazingly cheap. That's a rough estimate, of course. The overall effect is for the child to wear down his gift from grandpa from birth to age 21, paying $42 at age 40 to support his own grandchild. He pays for his own care from age 21 to 66. During the transition, a late starter would pay $200 a year for several years after age 40 to make up for his late start, and others would pay the same, but starting later. There are a hundred ways to do this, and the choice would be for the most palatable appearance. We have other, possibly more acceptable, approaches, but this one links well with other goals.

Proposal 22: Congress should enable one voluntary transfer between the Health Savings Accounts of members of the same family, especially grandparents and grandchildren, or one transfer to a general pool for atypical families. Members of the grandparent generation who have no grandchildren may choose one substitute from outside the family, or leave the decision to the fund.

Proposal 23: Congress should permit voluntary buy-outs from the Medicare program, which include consideration of returning payroll deductions, and fair accounting for premiums, copayments and benefits already paid for by age groups in transition; but make little effort to encourage buyouts, until prices start to fall.

All in all, the conclusion of this analysis is that targeted programs are probably better for the thirty million people with special needs, so universal one-size-fits all is probably not a good goal. Privatizing Medicare is a good goal, but we may not be quite ready for it. What's left is to fund the healthcare of children, by mildly overfunding the healthcare of seniors. That ought to end the discussion of this topic, except for demonstrating how you would control the money machine, exposed by the lack of a gold or other standard for the currency. It's done by bringing balances to zero once in a while, and it was uncovered by working around the grandparent-grandchild transfer. By studying what's left, we reach the conclusion that fixing the children problem would do the most good for the least cost, and just about everything else has major disadvantages.

Let us then do this much without waiting to see what Obamacare is going to do. If the Federal Reserve's inflation targeting serves the purpose, this may be held in reserve, but the failure of Keynesians to reach 2% inflation when they try to inflate on purpose, should make everyone uneasy about their approach in a currency system which depends on printing money until short-term interest rates rise to 2%. As the man in the audience called out, "Haven't you been to the grocery store, lately?"

That Dratted Third Rail

During all of the Obamacare uproar, I was giving speeches, and I can tell you that old folks didn't care a hoot, one way or the other. Obamacare wasn't going to affect their medical care at all, so they had only one passing concern. They were afraid Obamacare would cost so much, it would be necessary to raid Medicare to support the promises. As long as no one brought up that issue, retirees didn't care. But as soon as I tested them on the point, they uncoiled like a spring. Plenty of politicians saw the same phenomenon, and nick-named Medicare insurance reform "the Third Rail of Politics". Just touch it, and you're dead. The mathematics are already so strong, no mathematical argument is going to influence any opinion. Essentially, there's a way to make Medicare almost free, but it doesn't matter. What matters is if politics get ugly, political candidates will say almost anything. Right now, and for some time to come, nobody wants to listen to mathematical arguments. They want to know if a red-mouthed opponent can upset them at the polls, by using reckless attacks. They can, and will, and there isn't much that can be done about it. The consequence is, the easiest argument for using compound interest to pay for health insurance is to privatize Medicare, but it has the most political obstacles to overcome.

Whereas, using the same approach for younger people has difficult math because of the shorter time periods. But it has a much easier time of it politically, because young people often don't have insurance, or need insurance, and so they have very little to lose. Furthermore, the regulations issued for Obamacare were often selected for the purpose of hindering Heath Savings Accounts. Much of the coming battle in Congress will be fought over trenches and fences, seemingly erected for the purpose of making progress difficult. That will be true for more than Health Savings Accounts, but that fact is just another irrelevance.

Here's another unexpected twist which will influence future trends. When Medicare emerged from the sausage factory of legislative construction, the hospital part (Part A) was entirely funded by government subsidy, and therefore is an obvious target for adding revenue, based on the fairness argument. That tends to crowd this heavy expense into the category funded by something else, and makes the pressure stronger. By another quirk of legislation, Medicare is a subchapter of the Social Security Act, which is now starting to need revenue. So the mechanism already exists to merge retirement income with Medicare surplus, if we ever get a Medicare surplus. The doctor reimbursement part of the Act (Part B) is what people nominally pay for when they pay their Medicare premiums. Now, add the DRG squeeze into the mixture.

Seeing hospital revenue for inpatients squeezed by the DRG, the hospitals have responded by enlarging their outpatient areas and hiring practicing doctors to join their staff on salary. Naturally, the salaries are inflated to attract doctors, and although hospitals pay the higher salaries, there can be little doubt they would squeeze those inflated salaries if revenue got squeezed. Meanwhile, Medicare is confronted with a mass movement of doctors from Part B to Part A, and so it raises the premiums in extraordinary jumps, but that only affects the premium still more. Unless things are changed, that means there will be less money for Social Security, and the hope of merging the two programs will be greatly injured. Meanwhile, if the hospitals squeeze the salaries, there will be a surge of physician returnees to private practice, ultimately raising Part B premiums, or else lowering physician incomes, leading to a doctor shortage unless reimbursement is raised. Because this was all unexpected, some patchwork will be applied. But the long-run consequence will be a decreased likelihood of merging Social Security with Medicare, which I believe would be a bad consequence for health insurance design. What a tangled web we weave.

Half-Started HSAs

T here's another quirk in the law, which may or may not endure. You don't need a linked high-deductible insurance policy to withdraw money from an HSA, but you do need it, to deposit more money. If you take advantage of that, watch out for the rule that you can't have two government plans at once, including Obamacare,

Medicare, Medicaid and Veterans Health Benefits. So it's best to take out the HSA first, then the other insurance. This is such a complicated process, it might very well change, so be sure to ask before taking any action.

In any event, the suggestion seems valid at the moment, that the worst to happen to you is to acquire a tax-deductible account which you aren't entirely free to liquidate until you retire. And it has a health insurance feature which is also tax-deductible to the extent it has been funded, but which can be used to empty the account if you are strapped for money. If you have other sources of funds, it probably would be best to spend them first, since doubly-deductible health insurance is hard to find.

First Year of Life, and Tort Reform

The problems of paying for the healthcare costs of the first year of life are relatively small financially, but create large unexpected problems throughout heathcare payment design. According to CSS, the first year of life accounts for 3% of total lifetime costs, while all of childhood up to age 21 only totals 8%. By contrast, the Medicare age group accounts for 50% of costs. But the little tail is wagging the dog.

Without any prior earning capacity, pre-funding the 3% is out of the question unless Congress permits transfers of some sort from others. Legally, that means the parents, but the parents are usually pretty young and impecunious themselves. All manner of matrimonial tangles can occur, but even in the life of a blissful young couple, paying off that heavy cost may take several years to work around. It is hard to believe this issue would not delay the next pregnancy or even sometimes put it out of the question. There is little question younger mothers have a much easier obstetrical time of it than if they wait until they can afford the cost. The whole concept of a "valuable" baby was largely unknown seventy years ago. In my day as an intern, if a lady miscarried, well, just wait a couple of months and have another. The present generation of mothers are aghast at such callous attitudes, but that attitudinal shift is why we once had so many orphanages, and today have so few. The high cost of obstetrics must have something to do with it. We hear it said that women going to work caused a drop in the birth rate, but there is little doubt some of this was the reverse.

The employer-based system of health insurance has some advantages, and one of them is to create family-plan health insurance. Having now lived through two economic depressions, I can be pretty sure the present epidemic of fatherless children will somewhat subside as the economy recovers. But no doubt the traditional family structure has been permanently modified, so the residual will probably be felt as a decline of the popularity of family insurance. With only one poorly paid and overworked parent to support a pregnancy's cost, the burden is much increased.

Birth and death are nevertheless the two medical costs which no one can completely evade. Hospitals understand this as well as anyone else. So, responding to the pressures of high hospital ingredient costs, the hospital financial officer shifts costs toward obstetrical and terminal illness care or its surrogate markers. Cost accountants have to be careful, because if they shift it to indigents who pay nothing, they will be cost-shifting themselves out of business. But if they can somehow identify insured obstetrical patients, they shift vigorously, and the employer will end up paying for it. So we see the response of putting ultra-high prices on the services, drugs and equipment of the obstetrical unit, just in case somebody, or some insurance, might pay for them. Within a DRG system which permits a 2% profit margin on inpatients during a 2% inflation, a hospital administrator has to do a lot of tap-dancing around the obstetrical issue, and many hospitals have just abandoned the service entirely.

And finally, the trial lawyers. The trial bar has treated each wave of healthcare reform like Austrian soldiers at the Siege of Vienna – a failure to win any skirmish could lead to extermination of all their family, if not extinction of their civilization. Consequently, when lawyers hear talk of the concentration of malpractice lawsuits in obstetrics, they brace themselves for another charge of the tort reform Brigade. Any personal injury lawyer who reached this paragraph, needn't read more than five words to realize the bugle has blown, again. Slips and falls, and asbestos – be hanged, those doctors are now after obstetrics. That's right, I am, although the real legal culprit is found in excessive awards for pain and suffering. Elected judges have a hand in that part.

It took me years of working in medical economics to realize how destructive malpractice suits against obstetricians can be. Although 80% of suits are won by the defendant, it raises malpractice premiums to encounter a succession of nuisance suits which fail. It's been some time since I was active in the field, but at one time I was told 80% of obstetricians had been sued, and many annual premiums for obstetrician insurance were over $100,000 a year apiece. If that's no longer true I am sorry; but I have the impression it is still true. In Florida, recently, annual malpractice insurance premiums for obstetricians briefly went over $200,000

The closest I can come to a conciliatory explanation, is this. Some years ago, a state law was passed and widely imitated, to the effect that a plaintiff for a child should be given extra years after the age of 21 for the statute of limitations to run. If the time to prepare a case for a newborn is extended 25 years, it is probably not surprising that records will be lost by then, adverse witnesses will have died or lost their recollections, and so cases without living defense witnesses will be uncovered. Impecunious and therefore judgment-proof defendants may become prosperous during 25 passing years. The doctor may have retired and thus lost a reason for patients to avoid suing him. Or the patient may have become divorced and need the money. And so on. So I have a lawyerly proposal for a lawyerly issue. Malpractice insurance comes in two varieties, claims made, and occurrence. In both cases, the incident must have happened while the insurance was in force. In the occurrence policy, it does not matter when the claim was made. But in the claims-made policy, the insurance must still be in force when the claim is made. The loophole may be closed by purchasing additional "tail" insurance, but after a while, it gets dropped.

> **Proposal 24:** That a new form of "tail" insurance be devised for children and obstetrics, which covers economic damages but not "Pain and Suffering". Comment: the great majority of awards are not for economic damages, because that is generally covered by health insurance. The vast majority of spectacular awards are for pain and suffering, which cannot be measured, denied or remedied.

Proposal 25: That hospitals and others involved in cost accounting be encouraged to cost-shift the indirect costs of obstetrics, to other departments of a general hospital, to whatever extent is possible.

Grandpa Makes a Gift

A point which cannot be emphasized enough is that a Health Savings Account is just about the best way to invest, if you have given little thought to investing. The deposits are tax-deductible, and the withdrawals are tax-free if they are medical in nature. Even if they aren't medical, they can be anything at all after you reach 66. You probably ought to give a lot of thought and investigation to the particular agent you choose, because they aren't necessarily legal fiduciaries, no matter how friendly they may be. They have no obligation like a doctor or lawyer to put the client's interest ahead of their own, and they can later hire partners you don't care for, so make certain you can terminate the arrangement and switch to someone else without penalty.

Be careful to choose a representative carefully. But whether to choose an HSA, at any age and stage of advancement, always leads to the same answer: Yes, do it. That being the case, a certain number of HSA owners will find themselves with an account they don't know what to do with. There's almost always an exit strategy, although you may need professional advice to judge which one is best for you.

If you started your account near or after retirement, you may have the idea you will never have surplus funds. But if Congress can be persuaded to make it legal, one of your options might be to roll the surplus over to a grandchild or grandchild-like person. If this suits your situation, please notice that a newborn child has some special medical problems. In the first place, the first year of life is unusually expensive; in the aggregate, 3% of all medical expenses are spent on the first year of someone's life. To anticipate a little, 8% of health cost are spent before age 21, which is generally held to be the beginning of the earning period. Children are generally pretty robust, but when a child is sick, he is vulnerable to lasting disabilities of a very expensive sort, so you don't like to see a family cut corners on child care.

But newborns have no earning power, their future is in someone else's hands. The average woman has 2.1 children today, two women thus have 4.2. Four grandparents roughly have one apiece. The way the law of averages is working out, if every grandparent took care of the health costs of one grandchild, things would be close to solved. Things would have to be adjusted for the non-average case, but they would be close to being solved by adding one grandchild's cost to each average Medicare cost for the elderly.

In this case, however, the legal and political problems are greater than the financial ones, so it would suffice for a beginning, just to permit those who want to volunteer, to be permitted to leave unused leftovers in their HSA to children under the age of 21. If there is concern about dynasties and perpetuities, it might be left to the child's HSA, to be exhausted by age 21, or transferred to the HSA of a second child. The sum in question might be around $8000.

Random Suggestions for The New HSA

1. They could add twenty or more years to the opportunity for extending compound interest still further. That would be after a long buildup of compounding, which works best after forty years (see the graph). Compounding already introduces a 512-fold multiplier. Adding three more doublings would extend it to 4096 to one. You need this extra cushion, not for the ultimate result, but to get through a protracted transition. For this purpose, we might consider the 21st birthday – a moment of the lowest medical costs – to be the beginning of financial life. It would supplant the present obstetrical moment of the baby's ears emerging from the birth canal, which is the second most expensive moment in lifetime healthcare. This has its pros and cons.

2. Closing the inheritance loop would provide a social bridge between grandparent and grandchild generations, who until recently scarcely met each other. Therefore, we should avoid making transfers

completely automatic; to a certain extent, they should be earned. And there should be some latitude to modify them while money remains in the declining fund after the first year of life, for various contingencies. The new method of transfer provides surplus funds for the grandparent generation indirectly to overcome the heavy first year of life costs of their own child, seemingly by relieving medical costs for their grandchild. Other than that, there should be some latitude.

3. Since Medicare recipients are retired, there is a ready use for surplus funding to be used for retirement. Other alternative uses should be considered. Provision of a roll-over from HSA to IRA has already been enacted.

4. Eventually as science progresses, the Medicare population will contain most of the severe illnesses of life. If they get sick, they won't need so much retirement income. If they don't get sick, they will need the money to live on. If the transfer to a grandchild is made at death, the whole retirement issue disappears. Congress should consider whether it wishes to devote so much attention to this one issue, or whether it would be better to designate the Judiciary or an agency.

Summary. A childhood health insurance, linked to a health insurance for senior citizens, owned by two people linked by redefining a birthday or some other strategy, may well sound like a peculiar-looking idea. Using its surpluses for retirement, and also to fund the permanently unemployable, makes it look even more peculiar. But let me persuade the reader to do a little math. At 7%, there are 9 doublings in a 90 year life. 2, 4, 8, 16, 32, 64, 128, 256, 512. That's rounding up on 6.5% and 85 years, which are closer to realistic estimates of future longevity and interest rate return, but who can predict? Every dollar at birth (possibly redefined as the 21st birthday) is multiplied 512 times. Since lifetime healthcare costs are estimated by others to be $350,000 adjusted for 3% inflation, and half of that is attributed to Medicare costs, the grandparent would have to donate the sum of $350 at the child's birth to pay for all of Medicare, no payroll deduction, no premiums paid. That's a rough estimate, of course, and we still have to account for the notch caused by birth costs, and the gap created by age 21-66, now covered by Obamacare. Uncertainties about the legal status might reduce this to $70,000, which leads to the

$39,000 conservative promise. Restoration of age 21-66 might lead to a tripling of these estimated savings.

> **Proposal 22:** Congress should enable one voluntary transfer between the Health Savings Accounts of members of the same family, especially grandparents and grandchildren, and one transfer to a general pool for balances left over from the family transfer. Members of the grandparent generation who have no grandchildren may choose one substitute from outside the family.

> **Proposal 23:** Congress should permit voluntary buy-outs from the Medicare program, which include consideration of returning payroll deductions, and fair accounting for premiums, copayments and benefits already paid for, by age groups in transition.

Shocking News: N-HSA Doesn't Subsidize Poor People.

N-HSAs can expect criticism that they don't subsidize the poor. That is, the Affordable Care Act intended to include everybody, but circumstances made it impossible to cover thirty million people, like prisoners in custody, illegal immigrants, and mentally defective. In retrospect, it might be a better idea to design special programs for such outliers, since their needs are so unrelated. But even if they must be placed in a once-size fits-all program, it is complex to see where they would fit into a pre-funded program if they have no funds. Furthermore, children and elderly are themselves in need of subsidies from the working generation, so it is hard to see where to fit them in and still retain the architecture of the plan, without creating loopholes. These people were thought of as frequently underserved, not as the ones responsible for subsidizing others.

So it would be my proposal that the concept of subsidy be re-examined, such that it subsidizes recipients instead of intermediaries, that is, people instead of programs. That would permit such a funding agency to direct its payments to whatever the client designates, which would be an improvement, right there. It would encourage new programs to start up, and it would introduce competition to an area where monopoly is the more characteristic behavior. I'm afraid, however, that civil governments have not completely recovered from their contention with churches and civic organizations for control of private charity. Government has pretty well pre-empted this function, and political responses will still follow old patterns. It's worth discussing, but it is government itself which created this situation, and government is unlikely to surrender its victory.

Summary of N-HSA

In looking at what would be involved in launching full-scale New Health Savings Accounts (N-HSA) right away, we concluded there were too many obstacles to launching even a large-scale demonstration project with it as the centerpiece – unless it had some additions. That's based on the assumption it would serve those who are younger than 21, or older than 65. The underlying theory is almost certainly correct: we will in time cure enough diseases to make retirement living a more pressing financial issue than paying for early death and disease. But we aren't even in sight of the crisis yet, and many people still remain unconvinced it is the face of the future. So based on these assumptions, unfortunately this step toward a longer goal cannot be stripped of its survival features, even in the name of compromise.

In fact, we have not yet shifted disease to the point where important health costs are substantially all located in the Medicare age group, as plenty of defenders of the Affordable Care Act will protest, but which I contend is the next stage. The doctors who have received large cohorts of uninsured, such as those who work at Kaiser Permanente, are often astonished at how little complaining these previously uninsured people do. They have accepted untreated elective surgery as part of their life, and glumly submit to it. In a few years, we will work off this backlog of self-neglect, and there will be a great fuss about how much costs have come down. At least, that's what happened after 1966, and then we found rent-seekers taught us what a new normal looks like. This time, it probably won't take so long or cost so much.

Nor before that situation confronts us, will we be ready to look for things for retirees to do, and money to support them while they do it. But it will come, and it probably won't go away unless we think harder about it. My rumination is we should start with architects, to redesign more one-floor homes with home offices. Working at home isn't popular, but commuting is worse. Unless the storage battery problem is solved, and Silicon Valley gives us driverless cars. Everybody ought to have some sort of electronic hobby, which can be turned into a working skill after retirement. Amazon and Federal Express must foresee old folks working at home along with their colleagues in a virtual workshop. One thing is obvious; we will probably need the money we now spend on Medicare to supplement a part-time income. Although transforming Medicare, piece by piece into Social Security, sounds like a simplistic idea, someone had better think of something better before we abandon it. The Health Savings Account automatically turns into an Individual Retirement Account at age 66. Until a multitude of similar transformations are devised, we should resist disturbing that forerunner.

We have not yet cured cancer, the common cold, Alzheimer's disease, schizophrenia or Parkinson's Disorder, but when we do we must see a clear path toward pouring these savings into retirement income. And while we are about it, we must take what we learn and apply it to changing Social Security from defined benefit into defined contribution, with compound interest and passive investing working their magic on the idle money. But politicians have a different sense: not here, not now, when it would provoke hostility rather than appreciation. They won't change their minds until their constituents do.

The one concept which survives this reverie is transferring surplus wealth from the grandparent generation to the grandchildren, with compound interest in the meantime. That's an idea which can be applied immediately, even though interest rates are at an all-time low. When they recover, bondholders will suffer, but stockholders should enjoy a nice ride. It has been restrained for various reasons for decades, so it might just unleash unexpected results in terms of the birth rate, or the value of the currency, or other totally unexpected ways. But it's ready, even though retail stockbrokers, banks, insurance companies and financial advisors are definitely not ready.

Multi-Year, the Future of HSA

We've spent a lot of time on the 1980 version of Health Savings Accounts. It's already rolling along in action, with only a couple of suggested additions to make it better. The new 2015 version is also before you. But lifetime Health Savings Accounts are only a dream, to be worked on for months or years, because they invade so many turfs, and will require extensive legislation to become a reality.

It seems remarkable in retrospect it took me so long to think of extending "term" health insurance into lifetime multi-year health insurance. As the reader will notice, it rapidly expands to suggesting to some (probably astonished) life insurance companies that they take a look at the idea of doing the whole job, from investing to paying hospitals. Spreading in quite a different direction, it could expand to becoming a money machine which needs prudential restraint, even supervision by the Federal Reserve. Some of it may sound cockeyed, like putting a man on the moon, or a drone over the planet Pluto. But the reason it hasn't been tried has little to do with innovation. It relates to connecting health insurance to the place where you work. It's the employer who is reluctant to extend his involvement more than one year, because employees can be so mobile.

The required extra ingredients are pretty simple, since the central one of pouring left-over funds from one year into the succeeding year is already part of the classical Health Savings Account. The genie is out of the bottle, so to speak. It is highlighted that one-year term insurance primarily protects the insurance company, limiting its exposure to a single year. The investments are already pooled, and the many years of a lifetime can be covered by successive one-year catastrophic insurances, although lifetime catastrophic health insurance would be preferable, because it eases the "guaranteed renewable" issue. Tax exemption is already part of life insurance, but this tax exemption is sort of special. If the catastrophe to be covered is really a catastrophe, few people will experience more than one in a lifetime. But if you define a catastrophe as anything more than a thousand dollars, I'm afraid it is increasingly common.

About all the product needs is the willingness of the insurer to do it, and the willingness of government to permit it. When you do the numbers, however, you find that what then blocks it on a technical level is closing the loop, connecting the end of one life, back to the beginning of another.

This in turn is inhibited by the heavily borrowed healthcare costs of a child from birth to age 21, before he can earn a living. It's just about impossible to design a self-funded plan which begins with a $28,000 deficit. The rising costs from age 21 to 66 are quite suitable, but there just aren't enough years of compound interest to make the package viable. From where I sit, you can't have lifetime insurance unless you agree to pour funds from a different generation which has the money (and is willing to give it up or loan it) to cover that initial cost of being born. But if you concede that one point, oh, my, what a product you will have. I'm afraid that is unfortunate for poor people without a sponsor, although you will see how I do my best to work around that difficulty.

We started out with the difficulty of assembling enough money to do the job. With the notion of multi-generation involvement, we run into the reverse problem. There's if anything an excess of money-generation, mandating the addition of a limitation, which I would suggest is bringing the balance to zero after one grandchild has been funded. There should be no need for entanglement in the laws of perpetuities if the protection is built-in. I'm afraid I see no other feasible way to prefund any appreciable number of newborns, and getting over that particular hurdle is the main obstacle to lifetime health insurance. Otherwise, prolonged life expectancy would probably need to add another fifteen years to manage it.

SECOND FOREWORD (Whole-life Health Insurance)

T his second Foreword is a summary of a radically modified proposal. It cannot be implemented without further changes in the law, or at least some clarifications of the Affordable Care Act. To state the issue, it is that increasingly larger proportions of American lifetimes are not employed, and therefore are not able to take full advantage of an employer-based system. It becomes increasingly doubtful that thirty years of employment can sustain sixty years without earned income, if you include childhood. Further, there is every reason to expect further migration of illness out of the employable age group. And finally, while there are signs of reasonableness, the mandatory stance of Obamacare is not greatly different from a package of mandatory "benefits" imposed on all attempts at innovation before they can be tested. If changes in the law are required before implementation, liberalization might as well be in place before innovations are proposed. No private company could proceed at arm's length without advance assurances resembling cronyism. Everything else is negotiable, but the notion of mandatory pre-approval of any modification must be softened to something less sovereign.

Sickness itself has moved into the retiree age group, and will continue to migrate there. The means of payment cannot move from the employee group, so a two-step process is resorted to, with middle-man government controlling the flow of money between age groups. If we are ever to remove middle-man costs, this feature must be removed, as well. Meanwhile, the paraphernalia of medical care, the medical schools, hospitals and doctors, remain largely in the urban areas where employment formerly centered. So the government once more becomes a middle-man, and the system begins to resemble a virtual system, based on computer systems which do the job without actually moving. Until everyone stops moving, such duplication increases costs, degrades quality, and starts riots. We must move people less, and move money more. At one careless first glance, that sounds like shifting money between demographic groups, but picking winner and loser demography has repeatedly been shown to be too divisive; almost a prescription for a second Civil War. In short, we have fallen in love with a computerized virtual model, based on the faulty assumption that it is without cost. Here and there it might be tried experimentally, but it is far too early to make it mandatory. Consequently, it proves much easier to re-design the payment system, shifting money between different stages within individual lives, than to make everyone find a new doctor, just because the insurance compartment changed. It is absurd to make everyone move to Florida on his 66th birthday. Even redesigning transaction systems is not easy, but it is by far the easiest choice. Nevertheless, there is still too much friction in the various systems to make such improvements mandatory.

The best model to adopt is that of the university president who ordered a new quadrangle to be built without sidewalks. Only after the students had worn paths in the lawn along their favored routes to class, did he cover the paths with concrete sidewalks.

The issue at the moment is that money originates with employers, supporting the whole system, but their employees no longer get very sick. To reduce complaints, they are given benefits to spend which they really don't need, raising the cost of transferring the money to retirees who do need the money, but are covered by Medicare. We are in danger of repeating that whole cycle with Medicare, piously calling it a single payer system, when in fact it would be a single borrower system as long as the Chinese don't collapse. Expensive sickness now centers in the retirees, but within fifty years a dozen diseases will be conquered, and we will then need the Medicare money to pay for retirement living. Constructing massive systems without that vision will just make it harder to replace them. We are, in summary, in great need of a gigantic funds transfer system, since moving the people and institutions to match the funding is preposterous. But as long as the system has two champions (Medicare and the Employer-based system) in possession of all the money, we flirt with collapses in order to force rearrangements.

All of this is divisive, indeed. For years to come, the easiest thing to move around will be money. Eventually, institutions and clients can sort themselves out for geographical unity, and probably improved efficiency. But a financing system with the money for sickness in the hands of people who aren't sick, plus a governmental, system dedicated to an age group with almost all the coming sickness but unsustainable finances – is a wonder to behold. Therefore, we offer the Health Savings Account as having the flexibility to collect money from the young and healthy, invest it for decades, and use it for the same people when they get old. It can cross age barriers and follow illnesses, or it can remain with survivors and pay for their protracted retirement. If Medicare is modularized, it can supply the money to buy pieces as they begin to appear less desirable. It can redistribute subsidies to the poor if an agency gives it money, and it can adjust to changes in geography and science, since all it works with, is money. And it avoids redistribution politics by giving the same people, their own money.

For all these reasons, Health Savings Accounts on a lifetime or whole-life model seem the logical place to fix the broken vehicle, while we somehow keep its motor running. If successful, it will grow too big, so it should remain modular from the start. It has feelers in the insurance, finance and investment worlds. It could easily arrange branch offices for retail marketing and service. It should have networks for research and lobbying. But as long as it retains the branch concept and avoids the imperial one, it should manage to keep the doctors, patients and institutions functioning as the whole universe rearranges itself – at its own speed. The first major step in this process would be to clear up some regulations which did not anticipate it. With Classical HSA adjusted for interim role, the design stage can be undertaken to link the pieces of a person's health financing. Variations of lifetime Health Savings Accounts can be tried in demonstration projects, perhaps staying out of the way of the Affordable Care Act by unifying parts other than age 21 to 66, as the New Health Savings Account. And then seeing which version of lifetime HSA survives the squabbling. That isn't all. The really big picture is to absorb the pieces of Medicare, one by one, as sickness retreats from being the central cost, and the cost of retirement becomes the real threat.

Details of Lifetime Health Savings Accounts (L-HSA)

If we propose to adopt the whole-life model for Health Savings Accounts, then why don't we just add it as a new product for the companies who are already in the whole-life business? It's a good question, and most of the answer is I don't happen to own an insurance company. Somebody has to invest a pile of money to own one. You almost never hear of corporate pirates attempting a take-over, and many insurance companies make their profits on subscribers who drop their policies, although that's mostly term insurance. Come to think of it, these are mostly 19th Century organizations who sort of had the good luck to encounter windfall profits when subscribers lived longer than was necessary to break even, and then even kept living on some more. It isn't exactly the background of people who start new businesses with new ideas. Nevertheless, they do sell their products to young people, invest the premiums for many years, and eventually pay their bills to old folks, on time and cheerfully. And there would seem to be plenty of incentive. Aggregate retirement income fifty years from now will probably be many times as large as the present face value of insurance, and probably include a larger proportion of the population. They already have actuaries on their payroll who could do the math, and who yearn for the day a new product would give them a shot at being CEO. Like me, they have already had a look at the C-suite offices, and like me, compare them favorably with the Temple of Karmac.

"Who will run L-HSA, once it's legal?"

However, I don't know any of them personally, so the assumption must be made that L-HSA will grow out of companies that package C-HSA at present, and sort of have a term insurance point of view. Elements of it have been around for almost two centuries, but even the life insurance industry might become dubious to hear whole-life coverage of health insurance presented as an investment. As the level of income taxation rises, tax-free internal transfers assume new value, but resistance to higher taxes will grow. Extending life expectancy gives compound interest much longer to grow, it thus transforms what it can do. In addition, if you desire intergenerational cost shifting for health costs, you probably must incorporate some form of insurance as a pooled transfer vehicle. This combination also enables funds to shift within the account to a later time in life. It's a more attractive individual incentive for savings, than threateningly proposing your generation must support mine.

As a final feature, Catastrophic high-deductible is here added, providing stop-loss protection. Call it re-insurance if you prefer. It's single-purpose coverage, based on the idea that the higher the deductible, the lower the premium. So it follows that the longer you are a customer, the more catastrophic insurance you can afford. Cost saving runs through all multi-year ideas, but lifetime coverage is a cost-saving whopper, because of the way Aristotle discovered compound interest turns up at the far end. (By the way, that's why I suspect we have rules against perpetuities of inheritance.) It transforms Health Savings Accounts into a transfer vehicle for funds, from one end of life to the other, and must add debit-card health insurance for current expenses. Forward from the surplus of the present. And backwards from the compound interest of the future. The last-year-of life could be chosen as an example because the last year comes to 100% of us, and is usually the most expensive year in healthcare, not greatly different from the face value of life insurance. But needs differ, and a ton of money sounds pretty good at any age. A Health Savings Account can also be used as a substitute for day to day health insurance. Another synonym might be Whole-life Health Insurance, although multi-year health insurance is probably more precise. The idea behind presenting this concept piecemeal is to provide flexibility for both overfunding and underfunding, since the time periods for coverage can be so long (and the transitions so variable) that both eventualities would occur simultaneously to different individuals.

The simple idea is to generate compound investment income – not presently being collected – on currently unconsumed health insurance premiums. And eventually, to apply the profit to reducing the same individual's future premiums. Even I was then startled, to realize how much money it could save. It's a scaled-up version of what whole-life *life* insurance does for death benefits. Since lessened premiums generate greater income, the math is complicated even when the theory is simple, but every whole-life insurer has experience with smoothing it out. For example, if someone had deposited $20 in an HSA total market Index fund ninety years ago, it would now be worth $10,000, roughly the average present healthcare cost of the last year of life. Neither HSAs nor Index funds existed ninety years ago, and of course we cannot predict medical costs ninety years from now. This is only an example of the power of the concept, which we can be pretty certain would save a great deal of money, but skirts the guarantees about just how much.

There's one other advantage to using HSAs within the whole-life insurance model. It has always bothered me that life insurance tends to gravitate toward bond investments, matching fixed-income revenue with fixed-outgo expenses. But insurance companies largely support the bond market, which is many times as large as the stock market. In effect, their situation encourages them to increase the amount of leverage in the economic system, thereby increasing its volatility, and its tendency to experience black swans.

Furthermore, the insurance industry has accumulated a great many special tax preferences, based on the notion its social value is a good one. Placing life insurance in competition with non-insurance providers of the same services would justify extending the tax preferences to the others as well. The resulting competition would invigorate what has become a pretty stolid plodding citizen, with somewhat unique power over state legislatures. State legislatures in turn would benefit from increased competitive points of view among their lobbyists.

People would be expected to join at different ages, so the ones who join at birth in a given year have accumulated funds which would be matched by late-comers. In our example, if a person waited until age twenty (and most people would wait at least that long), he would need to deposit $78 – not $20 – to reach $10,000 at age 90. It's still within the means of almost anyone, but the train is pulling out of the station. Participation is voluntary, but no one saves any money by delaying, and learns a bitter lesson when he tries. Notice, however, no one pays extra for a pre-existing condition, either; it costs more to wait, but it does not cost more to get sick while you wait. If the government wants to pay a subsidy to someone, let the government do it. But nothing about the whole-life retirement system compels increased premiums for bad health, or justifies lower premiums for good health.

Whole-life health insurance takes advantage of the quirk that the biggest medical costs arise as people get older, and similarly health insurance premiums are collected early in life, when there is considerably less spending for health. The essence of this system is to reform the "pay as you go" flaw present in almost all health insurance. Like most Ponzi schemes, the new joiners do not pay for themselves, they pay for the costs of still-earlier subscribers, a system that will only work if the population grows steadily and/or prices rise. When the baby boomers bulge a generation, they bankrupt the system, but only when they themselves start to collect. Everybody knows that. What is less generally known is that "pay as you go" systems fail to collect interest on idle premium money; the HSA system does that, and it turns out to be a huge saving unless the Industrial Revolution stops. Medicare and similar systems don't collect interest during the many-year time gap between earlier premiums and later rendered service; potential compound interest is therefore lost because payroll deductions are used for other purposes. "Pay as you go" is only half of a cycle; adding a Health Savings Account converts it into a full cycle like whole life insurance, and furthermore returns the savings to the individual, rather than using them for insurance company purposes. Whole-life life insurance is more than a century old, but health insurance somehow got started without half of it, the half which could lower the premiums. Nobody stole those savings, they just weren't part of the gift.

All this creates an incentive to overfund the Health Savings Account. Surplus which remains after death is a contingency fund, probably useful for estate taxes or other purposes; but on the other hand the uncertainty of estate taxes creates an incentive not to overfund by much. Most people would watch this pretty carefully, and soon recognize the most advantageous approach of all would be to pay a lump sum at the beginning, at birth if possible. Before someone roars in outrage about the uninsured, let me say this would work for poor people with a subsidy, and it begins to look as though the Affordable Care Act won't work unless it is subsidized. In that case, a downward adjustment doesn't reduce premiums, it reduces the subsidy.

Investment. It seems best to confine the investments of a nation-wide scheme to index funds of a weighted average of the stocks of all U.S. companies above a certain size, and thus offering pooling for those who are (rightly) afraid of investing. This will disappoint the brokerage industry and the financial advisors, but it certainly is diversified, fluctuates with the United States economy, and has low management costs. In a sense, the individual gets a share in a nation-wide whole-life health insurance which substitutes long-run equities for conventional fixed income securities. It removes the temptation to speculate on what is certain to occur, but on dates which are uncertain. Treasury bonds might be added to the mix, but almost anything else is too politically vulnerable to political temptations. Even so, it will have downs as well as ups, and therefore participation must be voluntary to protect the index manager from political uproar when stocks go down, as from time to time they certainly will.

One danger seems almost certainly predictable. This book has chosen 6.5 percent assumed return, mostly because it happens to make examples easy to calculate. The actual required return is probably closer to 4% plus inflation. Supposing for example that 7 % is the right number, there is little doubt a steady investment return is only achieved on an average of constant volatility, sometimes returning 20% in some years, and sometimes declining as much or more in other years. Judging from past experience, there will be a temptation for some people to make withdrawals in years of bull markets, which could reduce average returns to 3 or 4 percent in bear market years, and fall short of the 7% average at the moment it is needed. In addition, the officers of Medicare are likely to be tempted to pay Medicare more than a 7% average in windfall years, leaving the running annual average to decline below 7%, just as the trust officers of pension funds once deluded themselves by temporary runs of bull markets. Ultimately this issue reduces itself to a question whether a temporary surplus is really temporary, and if not, whether the subscribers should benefit, or the insurance company. After that is decided, extending or contracting the accordion would get consideration. It seems much better to negotiate these philosophical questions of equity in advance, and establish firm rules before sharp temporary fluctuations are upon us.

Insuring the Uninsured. Because universal coverage has great appeal, I have gone through the exercise of calculating whether the impoverished uninsured might be included by using subsidy money to provide a lump sum advance premium on their behalf. It would work, in the sense it would be less costly, but I do not recommend beginning by including it. Reliable government sources have calculated that even after full implementation, the Affordable Care Act will leave 31 million people uninsured. That is, there are 11 million undocumented aliens, 7 million people in jail, and about 8 million people so mentally retarded or impaired, that it is unrealistic ever to expect them to be self-supporting. In my opinion, it is better to design four or five targeted special programs for these people, and keep their vicissitudes out of conventional insurance. Better, that is, than to include them in any universal scheme which the mind of man can devise. But to repeat, the mathematics are adequate to justify the opinion that it would save money to include them in this plan with a front-end subsidy of about five thousand dollars, adjusted backward for fund growth since birth. I refuse to quibble about investment size, since no one can be certain what either investments or medical science will do in the future. It seems much better to make annual recalculations for inflation and medical discoveries, <u>and then make adjustments through an accordion approach for coverage</u>. There seems to be no need to make precise predictions, since any benefit at all is an improvement over relying on taxpayer subsidies, which now run 50% for Medicare itself. This plan will help somewhat, no matter what the future brings, and as far as I can see, it would make the presently unmanageable financial difficulties, more manageable.

George Ross Fisher, M.D.

Converting Term Health Insurance Into Lifetime Health Insurance

W e start with the lucky circumstance that everyone has belonged to Medicare for half a century, and before that, large populations had Blue Cross and Blue Shield. The cost of healthcare at various ages is pretty well known for large populations. Since lifetime life insurance is cheaper than term life insurance, it is safe to assume lifetime health design is cheaper than year-to-year health insurance. The present inflexibility is one of the relics of an insurance system based on employer gifts to employees who are no longer as sickly as they once were. To go further, it also seems pretty safe to convert from a more expensive system to a cheaper one, and expect profits, except for the quirks of the tax laws. At the least, marketing costs should be reduced, provision would no longer be needed for gallbladder and cataract removals in people who have already had the surgery, and interest could be earned on unused premiums over long periods – if we could unify around patient insurance rather than yearly renewals based on place of employment. The system would become vastly more efficient, and interstate transfers would be facilitated. The methods employed by ERISA would be a good model for a start, and its experience would be useful.

> *"Accounting theory has it, every cost must be attached to a charge. So charges inflate to accommodate them."*
> **What Costs So Much?**

Whole-life insurance has its differences. Whole-life experiences fewer drop-outs, but makes an extra profit from investing the <u>unused</u> premium money for many more years. The additional investment income allows the premium to be lowered because it is not constantly threatened with non-renewal, and enhanced health care regularly creates greater longevity than the original estimate. So, whole-life insurance really can withstand careful investigation as a model. The bottom line is that healthcare would be less expensive if we shifted to the whole-life approach

This book's present proposal is to do roughly the same thing, converting term health insurance into lifetime health insurance, year by year. After all, that would start from a 15-million subscriber base. That's just the basic revenue source, however. Health insurance has a number of jumbled issues during a long transition period. The purpose of stressing the life insurance model first is to overcome a natural suspicion that we intend to claim magical powers of predicting the future. That risk is assumed to be stipulated, and we will not bore you with constantly repeating it.

Let's start at the far end, with the final answer to the test. In year 2000 dollars, the average American spends an average of $325,000 on health care in a lifetime. Women spend about 10% more than men. The main problem is to take a lump of money at the end, and restore it to different young people as they get sick. When they remain well, the problem of balance transfers is fairly simple. To insure the entire lives of 340 million Americans, the cost would be trillions of dollars. That's 110,500 trillions in fact, give or take a few trillion. Or 110 of whatever is one thousand times bigger than a trillion. The original mind-boggling figures were developed by Michigan Blue Cross from its own data and confirmed by several federal agencies; the future projections are my own. By the end of this book we will have suggested it should be possible – to cut that figure in half, without changing the medical part of it very much.

It is legitimate to be skeptical, since a ninety year lifetime history involves a great many diseases we don't see any more. They afflicted many people who would have been readily cured with present medications except the drugs weren't invented. As if that weren't complex enough, it also involves predictions about the health costs of people who are still alive, destined to be treated with drugs nobody has seen, yet. To hammer this last point home, it is roughly estimated that fifty percent of drugs now in use, were not available only <u>seven</u> years ago. Since we must go back ninety years to get data about the childhood illnesses of our presently oldest citizens, the unreliability of also looking ninety years forward from 2015 must be clear. And to do that for a population constantly in transition from very young to very old is daunting, indeed. But the facts of life, that people are born, go to school, get jobs, get sick, and then die – never change. What's new, is it takes longer to run the course, and thus opens up gaps between steps. If we gather the gaps and meanwhile charge premiums on the longer time intervals, we produce a brand new source of revenue. While the intricacies sound complicated, in the end we rely on going from a more expensive process to a cheaper one, assuming the transition costs can be supported.

The value of attempting it, is considerable. We already have a technique which the statistical community agrees is reasonable, which tells us lifetime insurance would require something over $350,000 per person. Future trends can be estimated well enough, to show whether costs-after-inflation are going up or down, and roughly by how much. A penny in 1913 money is called a dollar today, just for illustration. Naturally, we then assume a dollar today will be called 100 dollars, a century from now. Regardless of numbers games with the value of a dollar, we have a tool to estimate the general magnitude of health costs, and by how much they will likely change. It's useful, even when its answers are surprising.

Theoretically, there is room for a change in expectations. Some people may decide living eighty years is long enough, and then decline to pay for more. However, I've tried it, and I don't feel eighty is enough. So, for my own benefit if for no better reason, I decided to see what could be done with the cost problem. One solution is to work longer than retiring at age 65. If future medical care changes direction drastically, its payment system might also be forced to change. But if health care doesn't change much, the payment system won't need to predict the future. That reasoning reflects the insurance industry's own history, where the marketing department eventually asserts dominance over the actuaries, by declaring it is more important to predict generally, than with precision.

The approach has its limits. Health insurance did historically underestimate how much the payment system could warp the medical one over long periods, primarily because it initially mis-apprehended who its customers were. Payment methodology is now relentless in persuading its true customers, who are businessmen in the Human Relations departments of large corporations. They don't like to hear it phrased that way, but we now have a four-party system, not just a third party insurance, and its fourth-party directors, big employers. As corporate taxes rose, the system invented by Henry Kaiser in 1944 used corporate tax deductions to fund the third-party system with 60-cent dollars. In fairness to Mr. Kaiser, much of the system has migrated to take advantage of the tax deduction, and the tax rates themselves are higher.

Looking back over an expedient system designed for short-term goals, a shocked realization now begins to dawn: most current "reform" thinking is about how to twist the medical system to fit some unrelated budget. Even more shocking is the business customers discovered how modified tax laws could let them buy health insurance with a discounted business dollar. When donated to employees, another 15 or 20 cents could be clipped off. Obviously, if health insurance is subsidized by business tax deductions, and Medicare is 50% subsidized directly by tax infusion, health reform can't claim to be a reform until finance is fixed. Essentially, the employer-based system amounts to this: by giving health insurance instead of salary, the employer skips paying for extraneous things which have been linked to the salary level. Union domination of state legislatures has assisted this goal. Just for example, the Philadelphia wage tax is based on 4% of wages, the New Jersey income tax is based on wages, and so on. If you can find a way to pay the same, but claim the pay packet is smaller, you've got the idea.

Gradually we reach the point of rebellion; if it is legitimate for insurance executives to tell physicians how to practice medicine, it must of course be equally legitimate for physicians to re-design the payment system. So let's have a go at it.

Footnote: *In the thirty years since I wrote* <u>The Hospital That Ate Chicago</u> *about medical costs, the newspapers report physician reimbursement has progressively diminished from 19%, to 7% of total "healthcare" costs, so perhaps now it's legitimate for some related professions to answer a few cost questions, too*

As patient readers will gradually see, considerable extra money is already in the financial system, leaving difficult problems of how to get it out and spread it around. This isn't snake oil, or a mirage. The beneficiaries would scarcely see any difference in medical care if

Health Savings Accounts fulfilled their promise. But frankly, the insurance providers would have to make some wrenching changes. Since millions make their living from sticking with the present, it is undoubtedly harder to design a new system which would please them. We're not going to mention it further in this book, but the easiest way to remove big business from the equation, would be to eliminate the corporate income tax, and shift the tax to individual stockholders. It is not corporate <u>revenue</u> which finances the medical system, it is corporate <u>tax deduction,</u> largely because we have imposed a system of double taxation of corporate profits. Eliminate one of the taxes, and business might complain less about losing the tax deduction. Meanwhile, health insurers would have a new line of work offered to them. Corporate officers should, and often do, regard themselves as custodians of the capital in use, which in fact belongs to the shareholders.

What about the public? Well, medical care now costs 18% of Gross Domestic Product (GDP) and 18% is pretty surely crowding out other things the public might prefer to buy. In a sense, the political beauty of the premium-investment proposal we are about to unfold, lies in its primary aim of cutting net costs by only adding new revenue. Critics will say we pretend to lower costs by raising them. But essentially the money is spent to eliminate hidden subsidies and red tape which are off the books, and by other means which have been overlooked in the past.The accounting theory is that every cost must be attached to a charge, so charges have been inflated to accommodate that notion.

Better, but More Complicated: <u>Lifetime</u> HSAs.

Health Savings Accounts are a big improvement over traditional health insurance, and this book stands behind them – as is, without major adjustments. Go ahead and get one right now, regardless of what other coverage you have. Let me repeat: Their secret "economy" lies in keeping everyone spending insurance money as carefully as he would spend his own – but not being too dictatorial about it. No one washes a rental car, as the saying goes, so you can't act as if someone has committed a crime, just because he doesn't do everything for you. But just you let the individual keep what he saves, and millions of HSA owners will find ways by themselves to save up to 30% of traditional healthcare costs. HSAs provide an incentive for the medical consumer to shop more carefully, and consumers seem to respond. The difficulty is, some people are too sick to worry about rules. So, substitute a catastrophic high deductible for your present coverage if the law lets you do it (which is presently uncertain) but go ahead with a Health Savings Account and add to it when you can.

> *"Looking ahead to what might follow HSA, is one of the main reasons for doing it."*

In practice, the Savings Accounts (and their debit cards) are almost entirely used for out-patients, where an effective shopper can arrange a reduction in costs. For hospital bed patients there is no choice but to allow the hospital to set its own prices, except those prices must more fairly correspond to direct costs. Fair prices are mostly an accounting effort, concentrating on reducing indirect overhead cost attributions, with a few legal rules to ensure uniformity. But everyone must wait for that to resemble true costs more precisely, after indirect costs have been evaluated. Having repeated it all as a preamble, we now look ahead to how we might extend it to lifetime coverage, instead of the year-at- a-time variety. Looking ahead to what might follow it, is one of the hidden complexities of doing it.

One further simple idea: costs not prices. We have all assumed that catastrophic coverage is basic. If everybody ought to have something, he ought to have a very high deductible for a bare-bones indemnity policy. But just consider an addition: insurance for the health costs of the first year of life, plus the last year of life. That's technically simple to do retrospectively, although it takes most people a few moments to get it. And 100% of the population would receive both benefits, at a restrained cost by remaining uncertain just what the last year of life is, until it is too late to run up its cost. Indeed, transition costs would be minimized by eliminating the historical part of costs for the transitioning population, and phasing in the ongoing expense. Ask your friendly actuary; he'll get it, immediately.

Revised DRG coding and Methodology. Either way, if you guarantee to provide something for everyone, you better have a plan for controlling its boundaries. Inpatient costs affect patients too sick to argue about price, so hospital bed patients might as well be presented with some different options. They are more or less suitable for the DRG approach, but we have gone to some length to show what's wrong with the DRG coding methodology. The coding, among other things, must be fundamentally modified. As informed doctors will tell you, ICDA-11 isn't it.

DRGs ("Diagnosis Related Groups") are something Medicare started, which with more precise coding could be made ideal for the catastrophic insurance part of Health Savings Accounts. Medicare now contributes half of average hospital revenue, so its rules effectively dictate most other methods of hospital reimbursement. There are many problems with Medicare, but paradoxically, escalating inpatient cost is not one of them. Inpatient billing has been so muddled, most people do not realize that DRG has been a somewhat overly-effective rationing device. Like all rationing schemes it causes shortages, as inpatient care is shifted toward the outpatient area. Office and hospital outpatient costs are quite another matter, so the whole hospital accounting system has been turned on its ear. In particular, components of inpatient costs must be re-linked to identical outpatient charges, in the instances where they are really market-based. Then, a system of relative values needs to be applied to that base. For that, we will need a Google-like search engine for translating the doctor's exact words into more precise code.

> *"Single payer is not a solution, it is pouring gasoline on the flames."*

The Single-Payer Delusion. If the eyes glaze over at this endless complexity, take a moment to unveil this thing called single payer, which sounds as though it ought to be a great simplification. It's just Medicare for all ages, what could be better? Entirely too many people now spend their money on luxuries which they really can't afford. In a sense, the whole country plays make-believe that serious sickness is for old folks, who will be generously cared for, by Medicare. The facts are that Medicare is already running unsupportable budget deficits, and depends on foreigners to lend the money to pay for it. Extending that process to a lifetime of single payer is not a solution, it is pouring gasoline on the flames.

Furthermore, both catastrophic insurance and last year of life insurance are more similar than they sound. What most people don't appreciate is the risk of a catastrophic health cost is rather remote in any given year. But in a whole lifetime it is almost certain to happen at least once, which is often the last year of life. When you consider an entire lifetime, you cannot delude yourself it won't happen. Someone must plan for it, and the books must roughly balance.

Add Many Years to Lifetime Compound Income. Mathematically, it is fairly easy to show that healthcare costs will go down at the end of life; it's cheaper at 95 than at age 85. But that's probably a trick. We don't know what diseases will terminate life a century from now, so we can't count them. They are not cheaper, they are just unknown, and so we record the cost of the survivors of the race of life, not the average runner who will take time to catch up. If we are looking for lifetime healthcare revenue, recognize that practically all revenue is now generated by members of the working age 21-66. A lifetime system needs to extend its revenue even further to other lifetime age groups. It seems only right that everyone's longevity should be included, but laws may currently block the way.

It would help a lot to include the first 21 years, adding several doubling-time periods. It would also be useful to let HSAs run for a full lifetime instead of mandatory rolling-over to IRAs at 66. Obviously, the idea behind terminating at age 66, was that Medicare would take care of everyone's medical needs. But with time, Medicare has consistently run big deficits, to the point where it is 50% subsidized by competition with other federal funds, or by international borrowing. Adding forty years would multiply extra investment returns by four doublings at 6%, and at little cost to the government. This would be particularly useful during the transition, when many people start their Accounts at zero balance, but at a more advanced age. It would be a significant improvement to all these programs to end them with at least one optional alternative; terminating a health program at a fixed age is something to avoid.

Proposal 13: Health Savings accounts should include the option to be individual rather than family-oriented, and therefore should include an option to extend from the cradle to the grave, rather than age 21-66, as at present, and consider options for Medicare buy-out and transfers within families between accounts.

Permit Tax-free Inheritances of Funds Sufficient to Fund One Child's Healthcare to Age 21. In other words, we should make some sort of beginning to the knotty difficulty of making The State responsible for what used to be the family's responsibility. A second adjustment would recognize that essentially all children are dependent on their parents for healthcare support, until they themselves start to work. Children's health costs are relatively modest, except for costs associated with the first year of life, and the bulge would be even greater if insurance shared obstetrical costs better between mother and infant. Even as we now calculate it, the baby's health costs, from birth to age 21, are 8% of lifetime costs. A cost of 3% for the first year of life alone, makes lifetime investment revenue essentially impossible for many young families to support lifetime costs, because any balance would start from such a depleted level. So, the idea occurs that a considerable surplus appears when many people become older, if grandpa could effectively roll over enough of his surplus to one grandchild or designee. The average American woman has 2.1 children, so it comes close to a 1:1 ratio of children to grandparents. Young parents often have a big problem financing children, whereas in a funded system, the transfer from grandparents could be supported by a fraction of it, by application of compound interest.

With two statutory adjustments along these lines, financing of lifetime healthcare by its investment revenue becomes considerably easier.

Whole-life Health Savings Accounts.(WL-HSA) It has developed in my mind that **Lifetime Health Insurance** would become even better for cost savings, with the addition of one more feature, copied from life insurance, and combined with the needed DRG revision. It is, broadly, **the difference between one-year term life insurance, and whole-life insurance**, which offers lifetime coverage as a variant of multi-year coverage. Life insurance agents frequently argue that whole-life is much cheaper in the long run than term life insurance. What they may not tell you is that most of the apparent profitability of term insurance derives from so many people dropping their policies without collecting any benefits at all. Comparing apples with apples, whole-life insurance is not just cheaper, but vastly cheaper.

For those who don't understand, one-year term insurance covers illnesses for a single year, and then is open for renegotiation. By contrast, a whole life policy covers a lifetime of risk, overcharging young people for it in a certain sense, meanwhile investing the unused part for later years when health risks are greater. Does that start to sound familiar? The client is seemingly overcharged at first, but in the long run his lifetime insurance cost is far cheaper. Not just a little cheaper, but just a fraction of what a chain of yearly prices would cost.

It doesn't mean you must enroll at birth and remain insured until death; it means any multi-year insurance becomes cheaper, depending on the age you begin and the age you cash out – often at death but not necessarily. What makes the saving so astonishing is the way life expectancy has lengthened. We have been so uneasy about rising medical costs we didn't much notice that people were living thirty years longer than in 1900. As a rule of thumb money earning 7% will double in ten years; in thirty years, it become eight times as big. If you lose half of it in a stock market crash, you still end up with four times as much. This is what would be new about lifetime accounts, and it can be easily shown that overall savings for everyone would be more than anyone is likely to guess.

Let me interject an answer before the question is asked. Why can't the government do the same thing? And the answer is, maybe they could, except two hundred years of history have shown the American public is extremely averse to letting anyone be both a player and an umpire. For more than a century at first, there was a strong political suspicion of the government running a bank, or even borrowing money with bond issues. Yes, the government could invest in businesses, but we would then be guaranteed a century of rebellion if we tried to have government do, what any citizen is free to do on his own. Indeed, a review of Latin American history shows what disaster we have avoided by retaining this negative instinct to allowing the camel's nose under the tent. The separation of church and state is a similar example of how our success as a nation has been based on gut feelings. The separation of business and state is at least as fundamental as separating church and state. And for the same reason: we instinctively avoid having the umpire play on one of the teams.

> **Proposal 14:** Congress should authorize a new, lifetime, version of Health Savings Accounts, which includes annual rollover of accounts from any age, from cradle to grave, and conversion to an IRA at optional termination. Investments in this account are subject to special rules, designed to produce maximum safe passive total return, and limiting administrative overhead to a reasonable, competitive, amount. The account should be linked to a high-deductible catastrophic health insurance policy, with permanently guaranteed renewal, transferable at the client's annual option. The option should also be considered of linking the HSA to a policy for retrospective coverage of first year of life and last year of life, combined. These two years are disproportionately expensive, and they affect 100% of the population. Subtracting their costs from catastrophic coverage should greatly reduce catastrophic premiums.

Lifetime Health Savings Accounts (L-HSA) would differ from ordinary C-HSA in two major ways, and the first is obvious from the name. In addition to meeting each medical cost as it comes along, or at most managing each year's health costs, the lifetime Health Savings Account would try to project whole lifetimes of medical costs and make much greater use of compound income on long-term invested reserves. The concept seeks new ways to finance the whole bundle more efficiently, and one of them is health expenses are increasingly crowded toward the end of life, preceded by many years of good health, which build up individually unused reserves and earn income on them. Since the expanded proposal requires major legislation to make it work, it must be presented here in concept form only, for Congress to think about and possibly modify extensively. This proposal does not claim to be ready for immediate implementation. It is presented here to promote the necessary legal (and attitudinal) changes first needed to implement its value. And frankly, a change this large in 18% of GDP is better phased in gradually, starting with those who are adventurous. By the time the most timid among us have joined up, the transition will have become routine. As a first step, let's add another proposal for the present Congress to consider.

> **Proposal 15.** Tax-exempt Hospitals Should be Required to Accept the DRG method of payment for inpatients from any Insurer,

although the age-adjusted rates should be negotiable based on a percentage surcharge to Medicare rates. The DRG should be gradually restructured, using a reduced SNOMED code instead of enlarged ICDA code, and intended to be used as a search engine on hospital computers rather than printed look-up books, except for very common hospital diagnoses. Also to be considered for those who are too sick for arms-length negotiation of hospital costs, are uniform reimbursements among insurance carriers and individuals, and between inpatients and outpatients, including emergency rooms, as well as a major expansion of specificity in DRGs.

Overfunding and Pooling. Lifetime Health Savings Accounts, beside being multi-year rather than annual, are unique in a second way : they overfund their goal at first, **counting on mid-course corrections** to whittle down toward the somewhat secondary goal of precision – amounting to, "spending your last dime, on the last day of your life". To avoid surprising people with a funding shortfall after they retire, **we encourage deliberate over-estimates, to be cut down later and any surplus eventually added to retirement income**. For the same reason, it is important to have attractive ways for subscribers to spend surpluses, to blunt suspicions the surpluses might be confiscated if allowed to grow. An acknowledged goal of ending with more money than you need, runs somewhat against public instincts, and is only feasible if surpluses can be converted to pleasing alternatives.

Saving for yourself within individual accounts is more tolerable than saving for impersonal groups within pooled insurance categories, but probably must constantly defend itself against the administrative urge to pool. Pooling should only be permitted as a patient option, which creates an incentive to pay higher dividends for it. The menace of rising health cost at the end of life induces more tolerance of pooling in older people, whereas small early contributions compound more visibly if pooling is delayed. Young people must learn it gets cheaper if you don't spend it too soon. The overall design of Lifetime HSAs is to save more than seems needed, but provide generous alternative spending options, particularly the advantage of pooling later in life. Because it may be difficult to distinguish whether underfunded accounts were caused by bad luck or improvidence, the ability to "buy in" to a series of single-premium steps should both create penalties for tardy payment, as well as create incentive rewards for pooling them. This point should become clear after a few examples.

> **Proposal 16:** Where two groups (by age or other distinguishing features) can be identified as consistently in deficit or surplus – internal borrowing at reduced rates may be permitted between such groups. Borrowing for other purposes (such as transition costs) shall be by issuing special purpose bonds. These bonds may also be used to make multi-year intra-family gifts, such as grandparents for grandchildren, or children for elderly parents.

Smoothing Out the Curve. There is considerable difference between individual bad luck with health costs, and systematic mismatches between average costs of different age groups. Let's explain. An individual can have a bad auto accident and run up big bills; as much as possible, his age group should smooth out health costs by **pooling within the age cohort** to pay the bill. On the other hand, compound investment income sometimes favors one age group, while illnesses predominate in a different experience for another. It isn't bad luck which concentrates obstetrical and child care costs in a certain age range, it is biology. No amount of pooling within the age cohort can smooth out such a **systemic cost bulge**, so the reproductive age group will have to borrow money (collectively) from the non-reproductive ones. With a little thought, it can be seen that subsidies between age groups are actually more nearly fair, than subsidies based on marital status or gender preference, or even employers, who tend to hire different age groups in different industries. On the other hand, if interest-free borrowing between age cohorts is permitted, there must be some agency or special court to safeguard that particular feature from being gamed. All of these complexities are vexing because they introduce bureaucracy where none existed; it is simply a consequence of using individual ownership of accounts to attract deposits which nevertheless must occasionally be pooled later. Because these borrowings are mainly intended to smooth out awkward features of the plan, every effort should be made to avoid charging interest on these loans. However, if gaming of the system is part of the result, interest may have to be charged.

> **Proposal 17:** A reasonably small number of escrowed accounts within a funded account may be established for such purposes as may be necessary, particularly for transition and catastrophe funding.

Where escrowed accounts are established, both parties to an agreement must sign, for the designation to be enforceable.(2606)

Escrowed Subaccounts. Both Obamacare and Health Savings Accounts are presently expected to terminate when Medicare begins, at roughly age 65. Nevertheless, we are talking about lifetime coverage, where we have a rough calculation of the cost ($325,000) and the Medicare data is the most accurate set, against which to make validity comparisons. We want to start with $325,000 at the expected date of death, spend some of it in roughly 20 installments, and see how much is left for the earlier years of an average life. Then, we repeat the process in layers down to age 25, and hope the remainder comes out close to zero. There are several things missing from this, most notably how to get the money out of the fund, but let's start with this much, in isolation for the Medicare age bracket, age 65-85. We are going to assume a single-premium payment at age 65, which both life expectancy and inflation in the future will increase in a predictable manner, and changes in health and health care eventually reduce healthcare costs, not increase them. Not everyone would agree to the last assumption, but this is not the place to argue the point.

We know:

(a) The average cost of Medicare per year ($10,900).

(b) How many years the beneficiaries on average are in the age group (18).

(c) Therefore, we know how much of the $325,000 to set aside for Medicare ($196,200),

(d) And know how much a single premium at age 65 would have to be, in order to cover it. ($196,000 apiece)

(e) We thus know how much all the working-age groups (combined as age 25 to 65, 60% of the population) must set aside, in advance for their own health care costs, when they reach Medicare age ($196,000 apiece).

(f) And by subtraction therefore how much is left for personal healthcare within age 25 to 65 ($128,800).

(g) We can be pretty certain average Medicare costs will exceed those of anyone younger, setting a maximum cost for any age.

(h) All of this calculation ignores the payroll deductions for Medicare and premiums. Since this is nearly half of the cost, it changes the conclusions considerably, depending on how you treat these points. During the transition phase, several approaches may be necessary. Furthermore, the size of accumulated debt service is unknown, or what the alternative plans are, for it.

Shifts in age composition of the population produce large changes in total national costs, but should by themselves not change average individual costs. What they will do is increase the proportion of the population on Medicare, thereby paradoxically making both Obamacare and Health Savings Accounts relatively less expensive. Obamacare can calculate its future costs with the information provided so far. But the Health Savings Account must still adjust its future costs downward for whatever income is produced by investments. We don't yet know how much each working person must contribute each year, because we haven't, up to this point, yet offered an assumption about the interest rate they must produce. We should construct a table of the outcome of what seem like reasonably possible income results. There are four relevant outcomes to consider at each level: the high, the low, and the average. Plus, a comparison with what Obamacare would cost. But there are two Medicare cost compartments: the cost from age 25 to 64, and the cost from 65-85, advancing slowly toward a future life expectancy of 91-93. These two calculations are necessary for displaying the relative costs of Medicare and also Obamacare.

Children's Healthcare. Someone is sure to notice the apportionment for children is based on income rather than expenses. The formula can be adjusted to make that true for any age bracket, and a political decision must be made about where to apply an assessment if income is inadequate; we made it, here. We have repeatedly emphasized that if investment income does not match the revenue requirement, at least it supplies more money than would be there without it. Somewhat to our surprise, it comes pretty close, and we have exhausted our ability to supply more. Any further shortfalls must be addressed by more conventional methods of cost cutting, borrowing, or increased saving. In particular, attention is directed to the yearly deposit of $3300 from age 25-65, which is what the framers of the HSA enabling act set as a limit, somewhat arbitrarily.

Privatize Medicare? And finally but reluctantly, the figures include provision for phasing out Medicare, which everyone treats as a political third rail, untouchable. But gradually as I worked through this analysis, I came to the conclusion that uproar about medical costs would not likely come to an end, until the Medicare deficit was somehow addressed. I believe we cannot keep increasing the proportion of the population on Medicare, paying for it with fifty-cent dollars, and pretending the problem does not exist. So it certainly is possible to balance these books by continuing our present approach to Medicare. But it would be a sad opportunity, lost.

In summary, we have concocted a guess of the outer limit of what the American public is willing to afford for lifetime health coverage ($3300 per person per year, from age 26 to 65), and added an estimate of compound income of 8% from passive investing, to derive an estimate of how much we can afford. From that, we subtract the cost of privatizing Medicare if our politicians have the courage for that ($98,000 -196,000) and thus derive an estimate of how much is available for health care of the rest of the population ($128,000). Because of the longer time spans available for compound income, at 8% it would cost more out-of-pocket to finance the $128,000 than the $196,000; it would actually be financially better to include it. The non-investment cost, on average, would only be $ 148,000 per lifetime, for an expense which otherwise almost insurmountably crowds out everything else in the national budget. It might be $98,000 less because of Medicare payments, or it might prove to be more, depending on interest rates and scientific progress. Believe it or not, that could be a wide improvement over the present trajectory.

That's how it seems at first when you approach the topic of multi-year health insurance. But there are several exciting additions, when you really get into it. It plods along, and then it explodes.

Some Underlying Principles

C asualty insurance formerly contained a clause making it **noncancellable** and **guaranteed renewable.** Except for disability insurance, most insurance no longer has those contractual promises, but the better ones will still "stand by their product". Prices were too unstable to permit a continuation at the same price as a legally enforceable right. In 1945, the Henry Kaiser caper changed the whole nature of the relationship, at the end of which the employees walked away with no individual renewal right at all, but got really great benefits while they had them. That was not a good bargain. Without a right of renewal, there is no good way to make internal transfers from young healthy employees to aging sick ones. Apparently, labor and management felt it was more important to get something out of the situation than to come away empty-handed. Most of these negotiations were private, and there may have been unrevealed considerations.

> *"No individual renewal right, but really great benefits while they lasted."*
> **Bad Bargain**

But the one sure outcome of this turmoil was a young employee had no assurance of health insurance if he changed jobs, and no sure way of transferring surplus benefits to his later years, even after remaining within the same employer group for decades. Older employees were plainly getting more value for their health benefit, but young ones could not be sure they would stay around long enough to enjoy it. In retrospect, this may have been a driving force in the enactment of Medicare in 1965. Employees experienced "job lock", which definitely meant they could not take stored-up benefits to a new employer, or into retirement. Furthermore, casualty health insurance was gradually changed by employers donating the policy to the purchaser, so ownership of the policy migrated into the employer's hands. The employer had to change insurance companies for the whole employee group, or not at all, so slavery begat more slavery. The negotiated group rates naturally reflected this change. The business plan of health insurance does not differ greatly from automobile insurance:

Premiums are paid to an insurer at the beginning of the year; and at some time during that or subsequent years, the insurer uses the pooled money to pay the claims. In practice, there does exist one important difference between the two types of casualty insurance. Many auto insurance companies imply they hope to renew a policy if the premiums remain paid, but hardly any *health* insurance is "guaranteed renewable" in any sense. You can pay individual *health* insurance premiums for many years to the same insurer, but the insurer still reserves the right to drop you.

This largely unanticipated disadvantage grows out of the sponsorship of health insurance by employers, since applicant employees are in no position to put strings on a gift. Its hidden unpleasantness was emphasized when millions of people were recently dropped from long-standing policies which did not conform to the Affordable Care Act's regulations. Original motives and understandings became unprovable after the passage of time. One could, however, easily imagine employers felt they might acquire new duties by law, and were reluctant to stand behind unmeasurable ones. One could imagine the insurers were uncomfortable with the risk an employee might move to a new state, and because of the Tenth Amendment to the Constitution, be facing insurers with no duty to continue coverage. This ACA dilemma came about in an environment with so little competition, neither the employers nor the health insurer felt compelled to wander into unforeseeable conjectures.

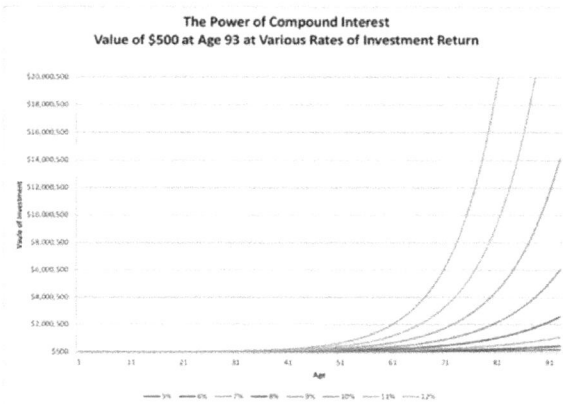

The Power of Compound Interest
Value of $500 at Age 93 at Various Rates of Investment Return

In this single subsequent event during the Obamacare confusion, a serious disadvantage of employer-based insurance discarded its tradition as harmless boiler-plate, revealing the enforceable facts of the matter. A health insurance company can unexpectedly walk away from an employer-based contract, even when it is needed most. The patient gets it as a gift and doesn't own it. This dispute over fairness and original intent was surely involved in the government's decision to delay implementation of Obamacare for large employer groups.

By contrast, we must point out the Health Savings Account leaves unspent money with the individual as permanently as he can restrain himself from spending it. For this he loses the ability to pool with others, and must buy high-deductible insurance to provide the pooling feature for large costs. Interest gathered on his idle money remains his alone. By retaining ownership in the hands of the employee, HSA gains protections against much broader health-finance risks, than the Affordable Care Act's pre-existing condition-exclusion does, for its population segment.

In fact, this sweeping violation of a gentleman's agreement may make such arrangements unacceptable in the future. If the employer community finds it impossible to live with guaranteed renewability, they may feel forced to drop the fringe benefit. Not everyone wants to exchange freedom of choice for freedom from the expense of it, but some do. Consequently, opening this can of worms could lead to dissolution of the present system, which depends heavily on the tax-deductibility of the gift for employers. There is essentially no difference between an individual income tax, and a corporate income tax, except the corporate tax is higher. The world's highest corporate tax necessarily creates the world's highest tax deductions for employers. Reduce their wage costs, and you will reduce their income tax. But reduce your own tax, and you reduce what it has been paying for. That's the bargain, and no stalling will change it.

> *"Some rude things it would not hurt to know."*

We must, however, introduce an observation which applies to all defined-contribution plans. The advantage has switched from the older "new hire" rather markedly toward the younger "new hire", because of the addition of investment income for the younger one. This is an advantage for one, not a disadvantage for the other, but negotiators seldom recognize such arguments. The terms of the agreement should probably be adjusted for this new development, which is illustrated in the first section of this book. But since the change is due to the mathematics rather than the judgment of the donor, experts will have to see what they can do about it, before it becomes a punching bag, desired by no one, but forced on everyone.

Employer-based health insurance was once a well-intentioned gift, with a regrettable lack of guaranteed renewability. Until the First World War, most corporations were controlled by founding families, and more employees enjoyed lifetime job security. The switch to stockholder control led to fewer benign gifts to lower-level employees. After a century of modification, the employee still is forced to bear the risk of losing his paid-for health insurance when he loses his job. The implicit good-faith guarantee of guaranteed renewability is however likely to vanish. Its implicit risk was transferred to the employee, but money to pay for it was not, until the Health Savings Account came along. With that, surprising discoveries emerged. Thirty years had been added to longevity, now making compounded interest money a truly substantial issue. Furthermore, many diseases had disappeared, generating overall a protracted interval of smaller expenses during working life.

As long as the (term insurance) risk of losing the premium flow remained, it was not prudent to invest the money in higher-paying assets, so the insurance intermediary was in no position to maximize float. Curiously, the famous Warren Buffett became one of the richest men on earth by buying entire auto insurance companies to transform the one-year "premium float" into a virtually permanent source of cash flow. Substituting health insurance for auto policies, essentially the same strategy is proposed by this book, for employees to consider. Except for Jimmy Hoffa, few unions have considered such a role, and in view of colorful union history, perhaps employers resist it.

Is there enough money in this approach? Some of the limitations to be encountered in paying for healthcare are specific and final; longevity would be one of them. At present, the average longevity at birth is 83. It would take some dramatic research discovery to extend it much beyond 93, but it is reasonably safe to project it will slowly rise from 83 to 93 during the next century. The medical costs of achieving such a goal are almost impossible to know in advance, but attempts are regularly made, and the best available estimate is $350,000 on average per lifetime, using year 2000 dollars. Women cost about 10% more than men, partly because of increased longevity, partly because of the statistical convention of attributing all obstetrical costs to the mother. There is reason to believe all late-developing diseases originate in the dozen genes residual in the mitochondria of the mother's cells, so the conquest of diabetes, cancer, Alzheimer's disease, Parkinson's disease, and arteriosclerosis – during the next century – is a reasonable prediction. Furthermore, new cures while generally expensive at first, eventually become cheap. Mix it all together, and while the costs of the next century may at times be towering, it seems entirely conceivable healthcare costs will become comfortably sustainable, a century from now. If we can generate the means to get to that point, give some of the credit to Warren Buffett, and John Bogle.

John Bogle may not have invented the idea you can't beat the index, but he certainly evangelized the news that 80% of mutual funds managed by experts, somehow don't beat the index. Let's explain. When you finally get over the idea of getting rich by out-performing the stock market, the idea reverses itself. The whole stock market is a proxy for the economy, and so although some people do get rich faster than the stock market grows, hardly anybody gets richer *in the stock market* without using some form of leverage, a genuinely risky approach. Professor Roger Ibbotson of Yale has compiled extensive data for the previous century, and convincingly demonstrated how relentlessly the American equity stock market has grown quite linearly, depending on asset class, but largely disregarding stock market crashes, and numerous wars, large or small. While small stocks have grown at a rate of 12.7%, blue chip stocks have consistently grown at about 11%. With big cheap computers we can see investors in stocks have received a return of 8%, paying a penalty for the small investor's inability to ride out really long-term volatility in any way but buy and hold. Perhaps, over time, we can find ways to narrow the overhead and return more than 8%. But for the time being one must be satisfied with 8% net, although 11% might become some ultimate goal. To go on, the 8% we get is made up of 3% inflation, so we better not count on more than 5% *actual* return. What will that achieve toward paying an average lifetime cost of $350,000?

The table plots how $400 will grow, starting at birth and ending at 83 and 93 years, with 5% compound interest. We've already described why 83, 93, and 5% were chosen, but why $400? It's a personal guess. It represents the amount I think would be achievable as a subsidy to "prime the pump". It might someday be a government subsidy for handicapped people who could never support themselves. And since it would be at birth, it would have to seem bearable to young parents. Many readers would react that $400 is too stingy, but politics is politics, and what people can afford is not the same as what they will vote to afford. In any event, we here are testing the math as a preliminary to announcing we can save a bundle of money by changing the system we are used to. Choose your own number, remembering we are attempting to reduce what is now reliably estimated as 18% of the Gross Domestic Product, and competing with a presidential proposal to give it to everyone. Further, the only thing you need to know about dynamic scoring is that making it free, will assuredly escalate its eventual true cost.

Compound interest always surprises people with its power, and in this example 5% just about makes the goal. There's not much room for error or contingencies. All of the known factors are conservatively estimated, and it passes the test. What isn't covered is the unknown factor, atom wars, a stock market collapse, an invasion from Mars. To be on the safe side, we had better not count on this approach to pay for all of health care. Just a big chunk, like 25%, seems entirely feasible. In the immediately following section, we examine the first "technical" problem. The first year of life is effectively as unaffordable as the last year of life, and newborns generally can't dip into savings.

Lifetime HSA and Whole Life Insurance: A Basic Difference

Over the years, much experience and lore has accumulated about running a life insurance company. Because the managers ordinarily are responsible to others who have risked private capital, more latitude can be extended to them than to taxpayer-owned entities. Consequently, it may be wise to obtain experienced counsel to suggest some business limits and latitudes which need to be authorized by law. The following is meant to suggest some areas which may need attention. And a lifetime Health Savings Account has at least one unique difference with whole-life insurance. A moment's thought about Lifetime Health Savings Accounts immediately highlights it. Life insurance has only one benefit claim, the death benefit. Once the flow of premiums begins, only one liability by a life insurer has to be made, the length and risk of individual longevity. The relationship goes on autopilot and a rough match can be made between the pool of bonds and the pool of policies at any time, adjusting only for policy additions and subtractions, or for fluctuations in the bond market. A Health Savings Account, on the other hand, must anticipate a possibly constant stream of deposits and withdrawals.

It is probably true, more money will be deposited in whole-life insurance in response to a fixed annual premium billing, than if deposits are optional in date and amount, so it probably would be wise for the manager of a lifetime Health Savings Account to calculate annually what deposit is needed, for each client to meet his goal, judged by his age and past progress. He should send reminder notices for the "suggested" amount. The purpose of health insurance is to provide money for healthcare when absolutely needed, building up a fund for potentially even more urgent future emergencies. We have partially surrendered the right to mandate the amount, in favor of creating incentives to save it. Consequently, there will be a more constant drain on the investment reserves, matched by a somewhat greater inflow needed from outside sources. The Law of Large

Numbers will smooth this out as it does with bank balances, but some volatility is unavoidable.

Since the general inclination is to limit the Catastrophic health coverage to hospitalizations, the attrition to their independent reserves in the account balance should be constrained (not limited) to paying at least one deductible, by adding one deductible to the escrow section, to reassure the hospital it is available. The non-escrowed balance would then more closely reflect the growing retirement savings earned by the arrangement. Since the Catastrophic Insurer is ordinarily an independent company, coordination is essential for long-term coverage. We can get more specific, but for now the risks to be managed are outpatient costs, less frequent but larger inpatient deductibles, and what for now we can call "all other". All three could usefully use reasonably independent escrows, which repeated display would encourage.

Overdrawn Claims. Since any client might be hit by a truck within a week of establishing an account, new customers present the biggest problem with getting escrowed reserves established. A large front-end payment can be required, and eligibility for benefits can be delayed. Lines of credit may have a place. Otherwise, established customers must fund and be compensated for the risk of early claims. Most organizations will probably elect some combination of the several approaches, with some combination of selecting which phase of the combined insurance should or should not subsidize the others, and how it should be repaid, and at what age. Bond issues are a possibility.

Overestimated Reserves. In the long run, solvency will depend on deliberate over-reserving, gradually reduced as experience accumulates. The basic premise is young people are comparatively healthy, whereas most of the heavy sickness costs will appear as the client approaches and attains retirement, many years later. Compound investment income will grow over time. There may be periods of mismatch between accumulating and invading reserves, so there should also be a provision for intergenerational borrowing and repayment, the size of which will be established at the onset. Every effort should be made to reduce these shortfalls by overestimating the need for them, possibly based on archived statistics from the term-insurance era. Nevertheless, future shortfalls and future bubbles will both be steadily predicable, and unexpectedly volatile, so over-reserving must be seen as permanently advisable. The consequence of all this is a continuing need for some allowable non-medical use of surpluses, such as conversion to retirement accounts, in order to generate reluctance to invade the reserves. The importance of this easily overlooked necessity, is very great.

> **Proposal 8:** Congress should state the principle that necessary Health Savings Account reserves should be somewhat overestimated at all times, linked to the incentive that individual non-medical uses of surpluses should be permitted at times when they are generally unneeded for health purposes.

Underestimated Reserves. And almost of equal importance is the need for early warning when reserves are threatening to become inadequate, in spite of every effort to overestimate them. Some sophisticated body must be created to oversee the growth of aggregated reserves, mandating increased contribution rates from subscribers. Since some subscribers could discover an increased contribution rate is a hardship, the oversight body must have the right to reduce benefits to uncooperative subscribers. That is, instead of reimbursing at 100% of cost, they may have to impose a seldom-used rate of less than that. In order to perform this unpopular task, the oversight body must have access to better information than the public does, to be in a position to impose small steps rather than big-steps. Under all these unpleasant circumstances, Congress could make the upper limit for contributions more flexible. At the moment, it is $3300 a year. However, while that amount now seems adequate enough, the figure is entirely arbitrary, probably set to prevent speculators from abusing the tax exemption. Therefore, if the upper limit is raised to address underestimated reserves, money might well be forthcoming to address the underestimate, which by then might have proved to be no underestimate at all.

> **Proposal 9:** Congress should authorize the Executive Branch to raise the upper annual limit for deposits to Health Savings Accounts, whenever (and for such time as) average HSA reserves fall below an advisable level.

Escrow Accounts for Future Needs.

One of the important advantages of Health Savings Accounts over historical health insurance lies in the contrasting sacrifices you must make if you can't afford everything. Traditional health insurance ("first dollar coverage") paid for the small things, but if you ran out of money, you had to sacrifice some big things. The Health Savings approach is to provide money for the big things first, and sacrifice little things if you must. That's the essential philosophy, and it has become exaggerated by increased longevity. We need to add a simple way to by-pass small expenses and save money for later. That's the reasoning behind adding escrow accounts to high-deductible insurance.

Think about it: when a subscriber faces a medical expense costing more than his account balance, he has three choices. He could forego the medical service, he could pay cash out of pocket, or he could borrow the money. Sometimes he will have enough money in the account, but saves it for some later purpose; in that case, he might be both a borrower and an investor at the same time. When it comes time to pay off his loans, that obligation should have a higher priority than investing new money, since otherwise the subscriber is investing on margin. Margin investing is generally a bad idea, but it can be made less risky through using an escrow account. That's a designated-purpose account, which is more difficult to invade. So, he may divide his account into three escrow accounts, and the managers may decide they need even more. It becomes inflexible if it can never be invaded, but it shouldn't be easy, and paying cash or tax-unsheltered money is always better if you can.

Borrowing Escrow. It's wise to pay off debts early, so the program should require its permission to do anything else with a new deposit. Not all managers of HSA will advance overdrafts, but some will, probably at rather high interest rates. More

> *"If you will need it later, Set it Aside, Now."*
> **Escrow Subaccounts**

commonly other subscribers will have surplus money they would like to lend like a credit union, because deposits up to their annual limit are tax deductible, and they would be reluctant to pay the taxes to redeem them.

It's possible to imagine gaming such arrangements of differing tax liability, so Congress must decide what circumstances permit it. With insurance, considerable pooling of resources happens without tax consequences, but when bank accounts are individually owned, pooling is not allowed without legal provision. Depositing unencumbered money in the escrow account is the same as investing it, except its presence indicates availability for loans in certain circumstances. Nevertheless, it is inevitable that gaps between the two curves, revenue and expense, will develop, even though the hills eventually exceed the valleys.

My suggestion is to limit structural borrowing at low interest rates to smoothing out the valleys characteristic of entire age levels, rather than provide individual banking arrangements between subscribers. Over time, these variations will standardize. And since the accounts will collectively grow, the quirks will eventually stabilize the investment accounts, possibly even augmenting income. However, if a surplus or deficit is exhausted, it should not be perpetuated with outside financing. The accounts operate under the principle that they come out right at the end. It therefore ought to be possible to adjust age-determined structural imbalances in bulk, while attempts by subscribers to game such variations should be countered by modifying interest rates. Wholesale buyouts have their advantages, but piecemeal buy-outs are better.

> **Proposal 5:** Congress is urged to permit pooling (at low interest) between the accounts of an age group in consistent surplus, – and other age groups in consistently deficit status, – occasioned by persistent divergences between revenue and medical withdrawals at differing ages. If there are other imbalances created by differential depositing, they should be corrected by adjusting internal interest rates. (2735)

Medicare Escrow. There are a number of reasons why some people would want to buy their way out of Medicare, whereas others would become terrified at any mention of changes in their Medicare plan. The incentive for the government to permit Medicare buy-outs would lie in ridding itself of its deficit financing, with secondary borrowing from foreign nations. And the advantage for the plan itself is providing a cushion for transition to lifetime accounts, ultimately a better cushion for revenue misjudgments.

By noting the average annual cost of Medicare, the number of Medicare beneficiaries, and the average longevity of subscribers, the average lifetime Medicare costs of Medicare can be calculated. Assuming inflation to affect both revenue and healthcare expenses equally, inflation is ignored. Then, with various compound investment assumptions, a range of future income can be estimated. All of this can be estimated as requiring a lump-sum payment of $60,000 at the 65th birthday in order to make a fair exchange for the Medicare entitlement, and guessed at $80,000, if accrued debts are serviced. However, the individual would have paid about half of that with previous payroll deductions during his working life (a quarter of the total), and by buying out of it at age 65, would be relieved of Medicare premiums which amount to another half of what is left, or quarter of the total cost. However, that complexity of description eventually leaves half of the total to be made up by Federal subsidy from the taxpayers because loans must be repaid. It's complicated, because every revenue source available has been tapped.

The biggest issue is foreign debt to be paid back for financing Medicare deficits in past years. Consequently, in order to put a stop to further borrowing, the buyout price must be raised. Obviously, if past debt is serviced, more contribution is needed. Unfortunately, information about prior indebtedness is not readily available, so the entirety is here guessed to require a single-payment premium of $80,000 at the 65th birthday, for a full Medicare buyout. If the entire Medicare program, past and present, is to be paid off, there very likely will have to be a tradeoff between increased revenue from HSA deposits and diminished service of foreign debts. As a guess, the elasticity of HSA revenue of $3350 per year, from age 26 to 66, has already more than reached its limit. For the moment, we have accepted the present Congressional limit, which was presumably rather arbitrary. While it is possible to imagine this arbitrary limit could be made to stretch to cover lifetime health costs, more likely it will only cover a portion. But to cover the Medicare unfunded debts of half the past century in addition to current costs, will require some new concept, as yet undevised, and a good deal more information than is presently public.

> **"All-other" Escrow.** It is difficult to foresee which escrows will prove so popular they will require limits, and which others will be so unattractive they will require minimums. Moreover, it can be anticipated some people will wish to use account surplus as an estate-planning tool, while others will have no estate. A provision in law directing the uses of account surplus at death may thus appeal to the majority of subscribers, but actually may be highly unsuitable for the majority. Therefore, while it seems harmless to provide a vehicle for such individualization, too much should not be expected of it.

To most readers, these sums will seem prodigious, and indeed they are. Few people at present are in a position to consider them. We can pray for some relief from scientists, from the economy, and from demographics, because downsizing Medicare is a growing requirement, provoking even more drastic remedies if we sweep it under the rug. We need, first, to make Medicare more modular, so it can be downsized in pieces, instead of all-or-none. In time, we need to downsize it and use the pieces to fund protracted retirement costs. The long-term goal, for the scientists, the politicians, and the patients, is to make it unnecessary to spend so much money on health. Beyond that, the funding of retirement has no logical limit. This long-term vision of our future must first become a commonplace in our culture, so we will seize every chance opportunity to advance it in fact.

Spending Rules—Same Purpose As Escrow Accounts

Useful features are buried in the spending-rule idea. A portfolio would never go to zero if spending is held below a certain level; an endowment on auto-pilot. This magic number was once 3%, now is thought to be 4%. In trust funds for irresponsible "trust fund babies", spending rules are particularly common. In taxable circumstances, it is a vexing complication for non-profit institutions that federal tax rules require minimum annual distributions of 5%, somewhat more than a taxable account can sustain indefinitely, at least according to present theory, and assuming present costs. Every effort should be made to reduce middle-man costs, and the present rate of progress is encouraging. As long as medical progress continues to depend on a top level of talent, efforts to attack the cost of care itself may prove counter-productive.

In my opinion, a spending rule is pretty much the same as a budget, and the same goals can be accomplished with an escrow account, permitting no expenditures at all until a certain date, and then only for a stated purpose. And furthermore, there can be several spending rules, just as there are several lines in a budget. There surely ought to be both a discretionary spending rule and an inflation spending rule, for example, since inflation is beyond citizen control. As a practical matter, planning will generally mean 5% discretionary, and 3% inflation, for a total of 8%. Until recently, it was generally assumed if the Federal Reserve instituted, or Congress mandated, an inflation target of 2%, it would mean 2% was dependable, because the Fed had unlimited power to print money. However, in 2015 the inflation rate is 1.5%, in spite of heroic efforts to use "Quantitative Easing" to bring it to 2% by buying two or more trillion dollars worth of bonds. Inflation has remained at 1.5%, resulting in much wringing of hands. So spending rules help establish responsibility for deviations.

It is not useful to engage in political arguments over why this is so, it must be adjusted for. The consequence is we have an Inflation Spending Rule of 3% and an actual inflation of 1.5%, leading to a national inflation surplus of 1.5%. If a Health Savings Account has an Inflation Spending Rule of 3% only because that is what we have seen in the past century, our inflation is 1.5% under budget, which could easily be misinterpreted as an extra 1.5% to spend. When we figure out what this means, we can puzzle what to do with it, but until that happens, no spending allowed. Another precaution would be to have two spending rules, totaling 8%, only 5% of which is actually spendable. If we create special escrow funds for buying out Medicare, or passing to our grandchildren – same thing.

> *"If you don't limit yourself, Others will limit you."*
> **Spending Rules**

In the case of Health Savings Accounts, a spending rule of 6.5% within an investment yielding a net of 9%, is a special case, but a good one. The central purpose of the whole HSA idea is to lower the effective cost of medical care, by generating funds to pay for it. The more income generated, the lower the effective price of medical care, so why impose a spending rule? In fact, a spending rule for an HSA does not reduce the income, it only delays the spending of it, because either the funding account gets exhausted by the time of death, or it is rolled over into an IRA. Either way, there is no final end to HSA spending, only postponements. When spending is postponed, it eventually earns more income; the ultimate effect is more availability for health care. If a cash shortage forces the HSA to curtail health spending, the bills must be paid from other sources, usually taxable ones. So even in this situation, there is more health spending power ultimately generated, but it is generated by not spending tax-sheltered money. It could even be argued that diseases later in life tend to be more serious. Indeed, if a spending rule is under consideration for an HSA, it could be voluntary as long as there is no way to game it. Unfortunately, that can lead to coercion for someone's own good, always a dubious idea.

If a portfolio generates 8% but only spends 5%, there's a safety factor of 3%, almost exactly matching the long-term effect of inflation. We hope moreover, the inflation issue is addressed by using the theory that inflation of expenses should match inflation of revenue, but you never can be sure of it. It is, in fact, more likely they won't match. A spending rule increases the power to shift surplus revenue to years of high medical cost, which will be later years, and will, by compounding, actually increase the total amount of it. This consequence is not necessarily obvious. The spending rule guards another easily forgotten thought: the purpose of an HSA is not to pay for every cent of health care. It is meant to pay for as much of it, as it can. It is likely, to invent an example, to encourage skipping cosmetic surgery, so there will be money enough for cancer surgery at a later time.

The purpose of this soliloquy is to justify the establishment of escrow accounts within Savings Accounts, to keep the fund from wandering from its purposes, or at least to recognize it early, if it does. There should be a Medicare buy-out escrow fund, with a suggested budget calculated to make it come out right. And a Grandparent's escrow fund, and Permanent Investment Escrow fund, budgeted to pay for a future lifetime of care, alerting the owner how much it is below budget. These escrow funds are intended to be flexible, but intended to serve their purpose. HSA Account managers are encouraged to use them, and to explain them. By making certain escrows mandatory and uniform, bigdata monitoring is facilitated. Other government access should be minimized.

Paying for the Healthcare of Children

I t has been said by others that eventually healthcare will shrink down to paying for the first year of life, and the last one. Right up to that final moment, medical payments must somehow evolve in two opposite directions. We might just as well imagine two complimentary payment systems immediately, because the two persisting methodologies could eventually conflict unless planned for. Paying in advance is fundamentally cheaper than paying after the service is rendered, because there is no potential for default in payment.

The two methods even result in different aggregate prices; in one case you pay to borrow, while in the other you get paid to loan the money. Dual systems are a fair amount of trouble; remember how long it took gasoline filling stations to adjust to credit cards versus cash. When gas prices eventually got high enough, they just charged everybody a single price, again. This isn't just lower middle-class stubbornness. Dual payment systems slow you down, and profit is generated from repeated rapid transactions. The buyer wants the goods and the seller wants the money. Profit comes from doing exchanges as fast and often as you can.

"The last year of life is more expensive, But the first year of life may cause more financial pain."

In a well-designed lifetime scheme, with balances successively transferred from one pidgeon-hole to another, it becomes possible to maintain a positive balance for years at a time (thereby reducing final prices, because the income from compound interest keeps rising toward its far end). That was a discovery of the ancient Greeks, but Benjamin Franklin seems like the only person to have noticed.

However, in real-life health costs, there is one intractable exception. Because obstetrics can be costly, particularly the high costs of prematurity and congenital abnormalities, the first year of life averages $10,500, or 3% of present total health costs. It therefore results in pricing which many young parents cannot afford, in spite of insurance overcharges to catch up later. And thereby a multi-year stretch of interest income is jumbled up, often lost entirely. It gets worse: childhood costs from birth to age 21 average 8% of lifetime healthcare. Please notice: Single-year term insurance premiums always rise to a much higher level than lifetime, or whole-life, premium costs, because internal float compounds in whole-life. Modern medicine has also resulted in rising lifetime costs, with only this one obstetrical exception. Someone surely would have figured this out, except excessive taxation of corporations created a motive not to notice the effect on tax exempted expenditures.

This problem obviously could be approached by borrowing or subsidizing. Someone might even envision a complicated process of transferring obstetrical costs to the grandparents for thirty-five years, then transferring the costs back to the parent generation. Since we are describing a cradle-to-grave scheme, it seems much better to imagine a single person's costs eventually becoming unified. Grandparents do in fact share continuous protoplasm with grandchildren, but before that was recognized, the courts had decided a new life begins when a baby's ears reach the sunlight. *Stare decisis* beats biology, almost every time. A society which already has a high divorce rate and a great deal of other family upheaval, probably feels better suited to the principle of "Every ship on its own bottom" – except for this financing issue. For childless couples and parentless children, some kind of pooling is possibly more appealing, and the complexities of modern life may eventually lead that way.

In the meantime, lawyers, who see a great deal of human weakness, are probably better suited to suggest a methodology for transferring average birth costs between generations, and back, although a voluntary process seems more flexible. It would seem grandparents are often most likely to be in a position to leave a few thousand dollars to grandchildren in their wills, and age thirty-five to forty seems the time when competing costs are at a lifetime low, making that the best time to pay it back.

Some grandparents are destitute however, and some parents are basketball stars. There are surely generalizations with many exceptions. The process is happily simplified by a birth rate of 2.1 children per couple, which is also 1:1 at the grandparent/grandchild level, and our Society has an unspoken wish to increase the birth rate if it could afford it. For legal default purposes, matrilineal rather than patrilineal descent may be more workable. But – if every grandparent willed an appropriate amount to some grandchild's account, it would work out (with a small balancing pool), creating a small incentive for the intermediate generation to have more children.

The answer to this dilemma probably lies in revising the estate-resolution process, making HSA-to-HSA transfers largely automatic within families, devising a common law of special exceptions and adjustments, and creating a pooling system for special cases which defy simple-minded equity. A large proportion of grandparents have a defined indisputable obligation, and a large proportion of grandchildren have an indisputable entitlement. The difficult problems reside in the exceptions, and require a Court of Equity to decide them. We leave it to others to fill in the details, because there could be many ways to accomplish this, and some people have strong preferences. The basics of this situation are the grandparents with surplus funds are likely to die later, but they are still likely to die, close to the age when newborns are appearing on the scene.

When you get down to it, the problem isn't hard if you want to solve it. By arranging lifetime deposits in advance, a large number of grandparents could die with an HSA surplus of appropriate size. A large number of children will be born without a standard-issue family and need the money. After the standard-issue cases have been automatically settled, these outliers can be referred to a Court of Equity charged with doing their best. After a few years of this, the results can be referred back to a Committee of Congress to revise the rules.

A basic fact stands out: most newborn children create a healthcare deficit averaging 8% of $350,000, or $29,000 by the time they reach age 21. Most young parents have difficulty funding so much, and so all lifetime schemes face failure unless something unconventional is done to help it. A dozen more or less legitimate objections can be imagined, but seem worth sacrificing to make lifetime healthcare supportable. The main alternative is to pour enormous sums into the government pool, and then redistribute them. I am uneasy about letting government get deeply mixed into something so personal. So, speaking as a great-grandfather myself, about all that leaves as a potential source of funds, is grandpa, and grandpas sometimes have an aversion to long hair and rock music.

Transitions To Donated HSAs, for Children

Let's proceed on the assumption Congress will authorize intergenerational transfers between HSA accounts, to the extent it becomes possible to create single payment accounts of the kind we have described. Presumably, most of these will be authorized in wills, but some donors may prefer to be alive when a transfer happens. It may happen at the birth of the child, or in anticipation of it; but accidents happen, so contingent plans should be allowed, with a default of some sort if this point has been neglected. If Congress authorizes these transactions, Congress should retain some control of them.

On the other hand, the child's parents retain fall-back responsibility too, and have a right to be represented in any changes. Congress should authorize a system of transition oversight, which includes state representation, and representation of parents, as well as experts with experience in related fields, like single-deposit annuities. The transition oversight committee (or court) should have a right to suggest technical and substantive amendments to the enabling legislation, have a right to hear appeals, and the right to obtain expert advice, and such other relevant duties as the enabling body may delegate.

Someone must be placed in charge of oversight over the amount of a single payment to start these accounts, adjust necessary supplements, and to adjust for any surplus. There must be an accounting system, and a public report of it. Experts in single-deposit annuities should be consulted, and future projections should be kept current. Since each year of life from birth to 21 years will eventually establish a "normal" budget, records should be maintained for the purpose of increasing or decreasing each year's average revenue assignment out of an overall children's budget. The purpose is estimating whether the overall budget needs adjustment, or whether only individual years do.

The presumption should be, the actual experience will be a near-zero balance at the 21st birthday. The possibility of surplus or deficit must be envisioned, however, and supplementation of the fund is preferred. However, if supplementation is not forthcoming, all payouts should be proportionally reduced to maintain a balanced budget. Supplements should then be sought from the parents of covered children, assuming such deficits cannot be maintained by transfers from funds intended for later ages of the recipients. It is not intended for fund sources for children born earlier or later to supplement deficits of other programs, although enough surplus should be generated to make lifetime funding possible. It should be recognized this is a sensitive point in the cycle, sometimes necessary as a brake, sometimes useful as a reserve. To use surplus to fund food stamps or agricultural subsidies is the beginning of the end.

The general principle should apply that a reimbursement agency should not be responsible for costs which were unknown before the revenue became fixed. In fairness, a new drug, instrument or procedure should not be reimbursed unless the next annual budget anticipated its existence. However, this accommodation should be reasonable, devoting more attention to the date of the annual opportunity to readjust the budget, than to political issues.

Here's the Deal

S o that's what I have to offer on Lifetime Health Savings Accounts. It's about as far as a physician ought to go in meddling in related professions. It looks to me as though creating lifetime accounts on a model of whole-life life insurance would be a great improvement over our present term insurance model. But I am quite uncertain whether a project this large should be monolithic or have competition between an organization with experience, like an existing life insurance company, an evolved version of one of our health insurance companies, or an entirely new organization formed for the purpose. This topic alone is worth a debate and a white paper. Several existing professions are involved and may have special legal obstacles, just as they would have special qualifications. Perhaps several demonstration projects should be launched to find out some answers before we get into a century-long, horrendously expensive, failure.

On the other hand, it would appear the financial savings would be too big to ignore. Because it would take ninety years to conduct a full experiment, it would appear fairly clear we ought to test this in component pieces and then figure out how to unify them. If we must make mistakes, let them be fairly early, drop them, and re-direct our efforts. By all means, ask the life insurance companies what their experiences were. How did they overcome the long testing period? What are the problems which term-insurance companies uncovered in their efforts?

In sum, we ought to spend a year debating the issue, several years testing likely solutions, and another year debating what we have learned. Only by following some such path, is there a chance we will end up with something we are proud of.

Health Savings Accounts
Condensed Summaries

•

SECTION SIX

Condensed Summaries

Summary and Synopsis

The Health Savings Account and its proposed additions endeavor to provide the following four most important benefits, which existing payment systems do not provide:

1. A system which encourages the subscriber to **keep the savings** he makes by letting him spend them, although it does not compel him to do so. It thus encourages frugal heathcare spending, with savings up to 30% of outpatient costs.

2. It allows him to overfund his health coverage, even up to $3350 per year, get a second tax exemption if he spends it on healthcare, and **keep the rest for retirement** income if he doesn't.

3. It provides a framework to take advantage of recently extended longevity, and recently improved investment methods, to **earn appreciable income from his savings**, with compound interest greatly magnifying them.

4. The only feature which is hard to explain is to **transfer funds across generations through reinsurance** rather than hospital cost-shifting ("Last year of life insurance"). At present, there is little public awareness of how dangerous it is to have one-third of the population with diminishing health costs of their own, supporting the other two-thirds who increasingly have most of the health costs. As this realization grows, this feature will seem more important than it presently does.

The key to all this, is to **relax the ties between health insurance and the place of employment**; the cooperation of business management and labor is essential to a peaceful transition.

This book suggests **two dozen other small reforms**. But if the public accepts the first three important goals, the fourth will come in time, and the rest are technicalities.

Simple Summary

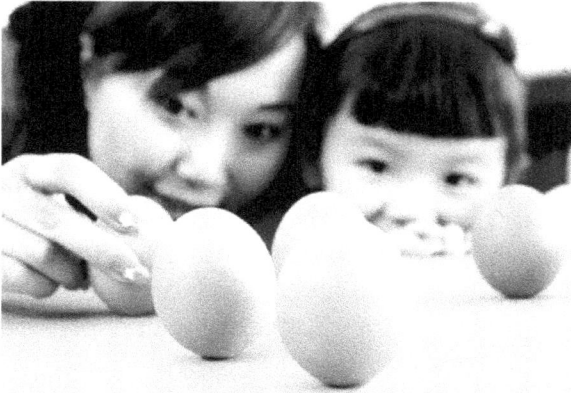

Columbus and the Egg

L et's summarize, in a slightly different way. We started with the classical Health Savings Account (C-HSA), which may need a little updating, but appeals to millions of frugal people as a simple way to avoid the tangles of present-day healthcare financing. The law hasn't changed much, but use by millions of subscribers has turned up many surprising features, all good ones. Deliberately overfunding them has unexpectedly useful results, for example, in providing retirement income if you have been lucky with your health.

On that foundation then was devised New Health Savings Accounts (N-HSA), combining six more innovations, each of which is easy to explain, but in combination utterly transform the basic design. The extended longevity of the 21st Century makes compound interest on passive investing into a powerful investment tool, and is used to reduce healthcare costs to the consumer, markedly. Secondly, improved healthcare for the working years has unbalanced the employer-based model, so sickness costs are getting crowded into retirement years. For this, the accounts permit extraction of the first year and last years of life, transferring their heavy costs to the working generation where employment-basing still makes sense. These complicated shifts may provoke suspicion until it is realized the cost would be almost imperceptible. And so on. With very little new legislation, most of this package is ready to go.

Lifetime Health Savings Accounts (L-HSA are patterned on a whole-life model. L-HSA won't work without some new legislation to edge around recent regulations and some outmoded premises. Multi-year coverage is cheaper, but requires a longer commitment, so it needs to be precisely designed. Starting fresh, it directly addresses a host of problems hiding behind a century of habit. Its flexibility accepts a range of designs, stretching from self-insurance out of a bank's safe deposit box, stretching all the way to letting life insurance companies run everything. What you find here are my ruminations on the subject. They are not definitive, they are just a beginning.

That's a summary of the health insurance part of this book. There's also a long section on the Hidden Economics of Healthcare, the kind even most doctors don't know much about, and the public knows almost nothing. Some doctors will even disagree violently, and either say it is biased, or decry washing our linen in public. At my age, there isn't much to worry about, so I feel the public will make better judgments about us, if they know some of it.

Summary: The Shifting Environment of Health Savings Accounts.

And yet another way to describe Health Savings Accounts, is as a series of places to put money, voluntarily moving from one category to another in response to the age of the owner, but potentially to environmental pressures. If the environment changes, the money might need to migrate, but it never disappears unless the owner spends it. Ideally, the money moves smoothly around in a circle, but it could pile up if some subscriber had unexpected personal situations. It's the subscriber's money, so we wanted to avoid locking him in, except by suggesting the most advantageous way to grow it or spend it. Many voluntary features could have been mandatory, with about the same result, but we wanted subscribers to innovate. The philosophy was that of the college president who built a new college without sidewalks. Only after the students had worn paths of choice in the lawn, did he order the paths to be covered with concrete. Here is a summary of the environmental factors we felt might change enough to warrant new pathways. The same idea applies to repairing the lawn after a hard summer.

Demographics. China found it didn't work to limit families to one child, and selective abortions in India caused the same disruptions. The baby boom bulge is a notorious example of a population bulge working its way through the steps, until it finally came to rest in Medicare, threatening the program with bankruptcy when later generations don't bulge enough to support their parents. Some bulges and shortfalls are predictable almost a century ahead, and while the migration of illness and good health is slower, it will pretty surely boil down to two enduring health costs: birth and death. So, the demographics of each generation are basic, and they are often predictable. In our society's view, there is little you could or should do about it, so although we can predict demographic surplus and shortage, we should accommodate the effects, not directly modify the cause.

Wars and Depressions; Inflation and Deflation. Major disasters affect all generations, but sickness concentrates by age. Furthermore, health disabilities from war affect those of military age and their successors, and recessions cast a long shadow over later income potentials. It might be helpful to set aside funds for these disasters, since it is possible to estimate the coming economic effects, and to start generating income for approaching shortages. There may even be usable information about earlier wars and recessions on which to base such estimates.

Economics is known as the dismal science, reflecting skepticism about the predictions of economists. However, they are getting better at prediction, and should be given a chance to estimate the future effects on health care costs, to the degree they modify the modifiers. The more we do this sort of thing, the more we may find certain predictions cancel each other out. And economists' predictions are likely to reinforce opinion that the best option is to steer for price stability, rather than resort to violent course reversals, a view not universally held by politicians.

The Nozzle of Transfer Points. It took the Federal Reserve a long period of experimentation to discover its most effective tool for modifying economics in the currency markets was to adjust short-term interest rates. In the economics of health care, I would venture the most effect can be had with the least commotion, by underlining the transfer limits as money flows between age groups. When the leverage at age 21 approaches over 500-fold, the ranges of power over health spending are enormous. Therefore, regular transfers from the federal Treasury may be quite small, but probably should be prevented from going to zero. Since it is envisioned that grandparents might bequeath a certain portion of their death surplus generated from Medicare without reducing Medicare benefits, the small initial cash deposit is a point which would be noticed least in a panic. Alternatively, adjustments of the amount the grandparent was allowed to bequeath could have a similar multiplier on far larger sums of money. Ultimately, such modifications would have to be reversed when such funds start to accumulate income, but considerable time would pass, between age 21 and 65, to accomplish it. Both government and subscriber must learn the cheapest time to pay bills is while they are small.

A second adjustment tool exists in the ability to require account balances to shrink or go to zero. The money would be given to the account holder, but would simply stop generating income until the required adjustment took place. Opportunities would appear at birth, at age 21, at age 65, and at death. Furthermore, large populations would achieve these ages at different times, so opportunities for adjustment would extend over a range of time. It took the Federal Reserve a long time to learn the sensitivity of adjusting interest rates, and it would take an equally long time to learn how to use these tools as well. It took a particularly long time to learn the most important lesson of all: what the limits were, for accomplishing anything worth-while with these tools, at all. Everything speaks in favor of establishing a monitoring agency, with defined powers and required limits, permanently devoted to this subject alone, periodically reporting its findings to the public.

HSA Proposals Summarized

T his book evolved while it was being written. It had to, because the implementation and judicial status of the Affordable Care Act kept changing. It primarily summarizes five proposed alternatives to that Act, all of them resting on variations of the Health Savings Account idea. They emerge in varying stages of readiness, but three are just about complete: (1) Classical HSAs, (2) The "grandparent" method of funding dependent children's health with compound interest, (3) The five-part proposal of the last chapter which begins with catastrophic coverage as basic, adds both-ends-of-life coverage to shift costs, and funds much of itself with compound interest. Two of the five proposals are expanded for discussion, but while cheaper, seemingly require too much transition time for present purposes (whole-life health insurance, and gradual Medicare buy-outs).

That summarizes the variants of Health Savings Accounts. The rest of the many proposals now summarized, either clear the way for the HSA variants, or else aim to correct some of the flaws in employer-based insurance. Not all of them are small and technical; the revision of the role of employers would involve a major change in the tax laws. And restructuring the DRG payment system would greatly revise the balance of power within hospitals. Inclusion of proposals on this list should not be taken to endorse a public sector approach over a private sector one. Nevertheless, many regulations do potentially stand in the way, so the way must be cleared. They are offered piecemeal because of different congressional committee jurisdictions. There has long been a question whether health insurance should be considered a health matter or an insurance matter, and the question is complicated by the Tenth Amendment making it appear the Federal Government is excluded from either activity. Special bond issues, might further complicate jurisdiction.

The proposals generally omit mention of their purposes, most of which are self-evident. However, each is accompanied by a citation number within the body of the book, where a fuller argument can usually be found

PROPOSALS FOR CLASSICAL HEALTH SAVINGS ACCOUNTS:

Proposal 8A: Health Savings Account Age Limits Should be Extended, from the Cradle to the Grave. The effect would be to create a continuous account, which could still grow over long periods of apparent inactivity.

One alternative option is to buy an American total stock index fund, order reinvested dividends, <u>take delivery</u>, and keep the certificate in a safe deposit box until needed decades later. (2718)

Proposal 1A: At present, Health Savings Accounts are limited to age 21-66. Provision should be made for inheritance of surplus to the accounts of newborn children and specified others, sufficient to cover their healthcare up to age 21, within a HSA of their own. (3320)

Proposal 2A: At present, contributions to Health Savings accounts are limited to $3300 per year, age 21 to 66. This should be changed to aggregate lifetime amounts, at least until latecomers have made adequate transition to the program. (3320) (2718)

Proposal 10A: Instead of the present annual limit of contributions to Health Savings Accounts of $3300 per year, Congress should permit a lifetime limit of $132,000 or more, with annual deposit limits adjustable to bring accounts at their present age, up to what they would have been if $3300 annually had been deposited since age 21. (2718)

Proposal 13A: Health Savings accounts should include more convenient options to be individual rather than family-oriented, and therefore should include an option to extend from the cradle to the grave, rather than age 21-66, as at present, and consider options for partial, gradual, Medicare buy-out, and transfers within families between accounts. (2606)

Proposal 3A: The annual limit of deposits to HSA should be increased by a COLA based on medical costs, rather than on the general cost of living. (3368)

Proposal 11A: Congress should reserve decisions to itself for changing the lifetime contribution level with technical amendments, and review final rules or appeals from contract terms which seem to threaten imminent, major adjustments to the general public lifestyle. (2718)

TAX-EXEMPT CATASTROPHIC COVERAGE

Proposal 6A: Congress should permit the individual's HSA-associated Catastrophic health insurance premiums to be paid, tax-exempt, by Health Savings Accounts, as long as present tax exemption for employer-based insurance is unmodified. This would make HSAs fully tax-exempt. (2687)

SUBSIDIES FOR POOR PEOPLE, NOT TO PROGRAMS FOR POOR PEOPLE

Proposal 7A: That health care subsidies be assigned to patients who need them, rather than attached specifically to one or another health program intermediary that serves them. (2687)

REVISED DIAGNOSIS RELATED GROUPS

Proposal 15A: As long as Medicare imposes DRG, tax-exempt hospitals should accept the DRG method of payment for inpatients from any Insurer, although the age-adjusted rates might be negotiable based on a percentage surcharge to Medicare rates. The DRG should be gradually restructured, using a reduced SNOMED code instead of enlarged ICDA code, and intended to be used as a search engine on hospital computers rather than printed look-up books. Also to be considered for those who are too sick for arms-length negotiation of hospital costs, are uniform reimbursements among insurance carriers and individuals, and between inpatients and outpatients, including emergency rooms, as well as a major expansion of specificity in DRGs. There is no medical advantage to limiting the number of diagnosis groups, and if there is an accounting advantage, a larger set is more easily translated into a smaller one – than the reverse. (2606)

COORDINATION WITH AFFORDABLE CARE ACT

Proposal 20A: The political parties would agree that both Catastrophic Health Insurance and Health Savings Accounts, singly or jointly, become specifically allowable options under the Affordable Care Act without age or occupational limits, and that all other interfering language in the Act or its regulations be removed. An appeal mechanism should be provided, not merely from judgments, but from regulations themselves. In particular, uniform tax deductibility is conferred by permitting health insurance and/or Catastrophic back-up coverage to be purchased by, or through, Health Savings Accounts. (3221)

COMPROMISE REMOVAL OF EMPLOYER-BASED TAX EXEMPTION

Proposal 4B: That a scheduled reduction of both the tax exemption of employer-based health insurance <u>and</u> the corporate income tax be prepared along the following lines: That in consultation with the Federal Reserve, the corporate income tax rate be reduced until it matches the average blended individual tax rate. <u>And</u> the tax exemption for employer-based health insurance be reduced in a step-wise fashion, until it disappears. The process shall take no longer than three (3) tax years, keep the two reductions in balance, and be reviewed by the Federal Reserve, and an appropriate committee of both House and Senate. (3106)

HEALTH SAVINGS ACCOUNT MONITORING AND RESEARCH AGENCY

Proposal 12C: Congress should create and fund a permanent Health Savings Account Monitoring and Research Agency. It should have representation from subscribers and providers of these instruments, with power to hold hearings and make recommendations about technical changes. It should meet jointly with the Senate Finance Committee and the Health Subcommittee of Ways and Means periodically. It should have extensive access to the appropriate Executive Branch department, to review current activity, detect changing trends, and recommend changes in regulations and laws related to the subject. On a temporary basis, it should oversee inter-cohort and outlier loans, leading to recommendations about the size and scope of inter-subscriber loan activity. At first, it might conduct the loan activity itself, with an eye toward eventually overseeing a commercial vendor. By this time,

Congress should be aware that it cannot cope with a program so large without an enlarged staff. (2718)

REVENUE SMOOTHING.

Proposal 16C: Where two groups (by age or other distinguishing features) can be identified as consistently in deficit or surplus – internal borrowing at reduced rates may be permitted between such groups. Borrowing for other purposes (such as transition costs) shall be by issuing special purpose bonds. These bonds may also be used to make multi-year intra-family gifts, such as grandparents for grandchildren, or children for elderly parents. (2606)(2735)

Proposal 18C: Congress is urged to permit pooling (at low interest) between the accounts of an age (or other) group in consistent surplus, – and other age groups in consistent deficit status, – occasioned by persistent divergences between revenue and medical withdrawals at different ages. If there are temporary imbalances created by differential depositing, they should be corrected by adjusting internal interest rates. (2735)

Proposal 17C: A reasonably small number of escrowed accounts within a funded account may be established for such purposes as may be necessary, particularly for transition and catastrophe funding. Where escrowed accounts are established, both parties to an agreement must agree, for the designation to be enforceable. (2606)

Proposal 19C: At this point, it probably would be wise to add some legislation clarifying the ground rules, if several professions would have to cooperate in allowing a new line of business for whole-life insurance, which seems a desirable outcome. (3277)

Proposal 25G: That hospitals and others involved in cost accounting be encouraged to cost-shift the indirect costs of obstetrics to other departments of a general hospital, to whatever extent is possible, to reduce the strain on the first year-of life, a constantly vulnerable point. (3255)

WHOLE-LIFE HEALTH SAVINGS ACCOUNTS.

Proposal 14D: Congress should authorize exploration of a new, lifetime, version of Health Savings Accounts, which includes annual rollover of accounts from any age, from cradle to grave, and conversion to an IRA at any termination. The model would be whole-life insurance instead of term insurance. Investments in this account are subject to special rules, designed to produce maximum safe passive total return, and limiting administrative overhead to a reasonable, competitive, amount. The account should be linked to a high-deductible catastrophic health insurance policy, with permanently guaranteed renewal, and be transferable at the client's annual option. The option should also be considered of linking the HSA to a policy for retrospective coverage of first year of life and last year of life, combined. (2606)

DIAGNOSIS-RELATED GROUPS PROJECT

Proposal 5E: Congress should be asked to commission a computer program to translate English language diagnoses into SNOMED code, preferably by voice translation. Suggested format: a search engine where English variants of discharge diagnoses are entered, and a SNOMED code number returned, along the general lines of – entering common phrases into Google and receiving file location numbers in return, except it would return the SNOMED code. If the code is not found, the computer accepts a manual entry by a trained person. Verified by an expert over the Internet to become officially entered into a master list which is periodically circulated as an update. The search program and its supplements should be produced on DVD disks to be used on hospital record room computers by other professional users. It should provide "hooks" so the Snomed codes and patient identification can be readily transferred electronically to related programs, such as payment codes and billing. (2634)

GRANDPARENT ROLLOVER SYSTEM.

All children are dependents of their parents, and the heavy costs of obstetrics (magnified by the unusual concentration of malpractice claims) make it impossible to devise pre-funding schemes. Young parents are often strapped for funds, so the lack of pre-funding is a growing problem in a Society uncertain of its family structures. Therefore, we have devised the grandparent roll-over. Tort reform would improve but not eliminate this work-around. (3252)

Proposal 24G: That a new form of "tail" insurance be devised for children and obstetrics, which covers economic damages but not "Pain and Suffering". Comment: the great majority of awards are not for economic damages, because that is generally covered by health insurance. The vast majority of spectacular awards are for pain and suffering, which cannot be measured, denied or remedied. (3255)

Proposal 23G: Congress should enable one voluntary transfer initiated per person between the Health Savings Accounts of members of the same family, especially grandparents and grandchildren, and one transfer to a general pool for balances left over from the family transfer. Members of the grandparent generation who have no grandchildren may choose one substitute from outside the family. (3254)

VOLUNTARY MEDICARE BUY-OUT OPTION

Proposal 22G: Congress should study the practicality of modularizing Medicare, in order to facilitate gradual buyouts. Voluntary buy-outs from the Medicare program might become desirable if Medicare costs should fall as a result of scientific progress, and religious exemptions are already desirable for a few. Consideration should be given to: returning payroll deductions, and fair accounting for premiums, copayments and benefits already paid for by age groups in transition, as early candidates for study. (3254)

BASIC INSURANCE FOR HEALTH SAVINGS ACCOUNTS, (AND OTHERS,TOO.) TRI-CHALLENGE BASIC COVERAGE.

Proposal 25G: Combine the high cost of the first year of life with the very high-cost last year of life, as the basic foundation of minimum health insurance.

It would undeniably be universal. What I am technically trying to achieve, is to combine one life situation, which sometimes generates surplus it can't use, with another situation, where every baby creates a difficult debt for someone else to pay. And whereas 100% of the population experiences birth and life at the two ends of life, there are societal constraints about sharing liabilities outside of families which must be explored.

Proposal 25I: And then, add Catastrophic coverage regardless of age, less the cost of overlaps. Title for the Package: Tri-Challenge Basic Coverage. (2882)

We thus design the basic benefit package to include two universally-unavoidable costs, plus the universally-inescapable risk of unpayable health costs at any age. It does not include any named service benefits. It is clearly superior to less universal, and more unaffordable, coverages. (2882)

Proposal 25H: Require the necessary coverage to age 21 for one grandchild per grandparent to be transferred between HSAs at grandparent's death or earlier option. Grandparent need not have a Health Savings Account, but must assure the required transfer amount, and grandchild must have an HSA to accommodate the gift. Probably it would go to a designated grandchild by inheritance, or to a designated pool of unassigned third-generation recipients – either without grandparents, or from large families. (2882)

This childhood feature adds about $28,000 to the cost of needed coverage, but because a century of compound investment income intervenes it would only require $42 at the child's birth to his death to fund the succeeding generation. (Added of course to the other two premiums, at 6.5% interest compounded from one year of age). The transferred sum at birth would have a declining balance and be entirely consumed by the 21st birthday. Because transition at grandparent age 42 (for example) would require $400 one-time contribution to catch up with late enrollment, rising to $28,000 for someone aged 65, it might be better during the transition to assess $200 a year for three years to latecomers, so as to reduce the even greater cost of even later joiners (over age 40) to the plan.

The latest of latecomers must be enticed, however, because they are the ones closest to activating the transfers, and hence represent the most important support to enlist to an innovation. That $28,000 seems like a high figure, and should also be investigated. Although it is only one of three cost components, paying for children is the most stubborn one, requiring the greatest contortion to resolve. The cost of the last year of life can be obtained from Medicare, and although the premium of Catastrophic coverage will vary with the deductible, its costs have been well worked out in the past.

The plan is not entirely complete: it offers the three components of the benefit package, the intergenerational funding mechanism, the HSA transfer mechanism, and the passive investment concept. How they are linked together is negotiable.

Its two important uncertainties are the size of the deductible, and the net investor return on investment in index funds.

Proposal 25I: This is voluntary Tri-Challenge Basic Coverage. Whether to make it mandatory, whether to subsidize it for the poor, and whether to replace Obamacare with it – are political decisions, not questions of insurance design. (2882)

What I Have Learned (1)

T his book has been an education for its author. Ordinarily, an author starts with a general principle, and offers a specific example of how it works. But I repeatedly found this field changed so quickly, changes in the numbers made the example seem awkward, if not invalid. Or one component changed, and balancing numbers were unobtainable. But I believe the underlying principles remain valid. It's better to earn interest on idle money than not to earn it, for example. But when the circumstances shift, the <u>amount</u> of interest to be earned – and consequently the proportion of healthcare costs it will cover – also shifts, allowing opponents to bring the underlying principle into doubt. When this process repeatedly leads to rewriting a whole book before it can be published, it essentially stifles debate. So I finally decided it was better to open the debate than worry about ridicule from hired political consultants over "framing the question", or protecting my offended feelings. At my age, what would I care about that, for heaven's sake?

So let's follow the trail of the book, and put together what I think I have learned, in the order in which it appears.

Pay for important things, first. Health insurance began a century ago, with good motives, but the wrong approach. It's upside down, in the sense that it started with the problems of poor people, and extended the approach to non-poor ones. Consequently, it offered "first dollar coverage" but threatened savings running out for truly expensive items, life-threatening ones. The most suitable way to get around this seems to be to have a high-deductible policy, which lets the patient decide what is truly most important. But two things then come in conflict: the higher the deductible, the lower the premium. That's good, but what's bad is the higher the deductible, the fewer people can afford it. So the Health Savings Account addressed this dilemma by linking high-deductible ("catastrophic") insurance to a tax-deductible savings account. In effect, the poor person could build up the deductible on time payments. It isn't perfect, but it was enough better so 15 million people adopted it, and their premiums became 30% lower. And so, more people could afford it.

Earn interest on savings. Then the patients taught me a lesson. In spite of abnormally low interest rates, people seemed to perceive that major illnesses come late in life, and longevity had lengthened considerably this century. And they liked the ability to judge their own health, letting the healthy ones pick stock investments if they chose to, because low interest rates shift many investors from bonds to stocks, which then rise. Sickly people could choose bonds, or tax-exempt savings accounts. Quite unique to American retirement funds, this one gave a second tax deduction when you spent it (if you spent it on health).

If there is money left over, you get to keep it. Conventional health insurance spent any left-over money to reduce premiums, they claimed. This one gave any money you saved back to you, as an incentive to be frugal. I suspect some people thought a bird in the hand was worth two in the bush, which means they didn't exactly trust insurance companies to lower premiums fully, but might have raised the salaries of insurance executives with some of the savings.

In time it developed a different significance: if you were lucky and healthy, you could spend the left-overs at age 66, for retirement income. The news about the approaching insolvency of Social Security encouraged that choice. At least, it began to look as though Social Security benefits might not be raised, so you might need the money more at a later time; compound interest made Health Savings Accounts worth more, later. Frugality early, led to more income later.

If anybody gets a tax deduction, everybody wants the same. For eighty years, employees of corporations got health insurance with a tax exemption, but half of the population didn't. That amounts yearly to a couple thousand dollars for a family, twice that much for the corporation itself (at its higher tax rates), and the possibility that even more escapes to foreign tax havens. By simply allowing the Health Savings Account to buy the catastrophic insurance which is required, this egregious inequity would disappear. If that gets blocked in Congress, then simply reduce the corporate tax rate, which corporations don't pay anyway because of the tax deduction. You might appear to be rewarding corporations, but you are really only shifting their deduction.

Save your deductions for later. It was a surprise to find 40% of subscribers to Health Savings Accounts paid for small health expenses out of pocket rather than take the tax deduction. It suddenly made sense that if the account would grow, and in any event you would get it back at age 66, you should pay out of pocket when it is small, saving the deduction until later when it had grown.

Split the payment system. Cash for outpatients, insurance for helpless inpatients. When you take away someone's clothes, and he is too sick in the hospital to argue, competitive prices are meaningless to him. Prices should be set by outpatients, who are free to trade elsewhere. A surprising number of inpatient services are identical to outpatient services, which should set the price for both. Some are unique, so a relative-value scale should be constructed to include them in the relationship.

Both the DRG system and co-payments are abominations. Payment by diagnosis is akin to service benefits, wrapped in a rationing system. Pay a fair fee for a necessary service, don't pay for an unnecessary one. As for copayment, it simplifies collective bargaining, but it creates two insurances for one service, and has been repeatedly shown to have no deterrence value.

Reverse the Maricopa Decision, preferably with legislation. Mrs. Clinton's plan of ten years ago was for a system of Health Maintenance Organizations (HMO). She can thank her lucky stars it didn't pass, because the public rejected them. HMOs were in fact invented by groups of doctors, and worked quite well. The essence of why they didn't work lies in the Maricopa decision that doctors were forbidden to run them. The Maricopa decision (4/3 on the Supreme Court) was based on a motion for summary judgment and never had a trial of the facts. Let's see if Congress can improve on that.

Substitute Catastrophic health insurance for any and all versions of limited benefits, including the Affordable Care Act. Catastrophic insurance is now privately run, and it is difficult to obtain data on costs and expenses. No doubt the plans vary considerably. But the system of indemnity insurance is superior to that of service benefits, and high deductible is superior to mandatory benefits. Catastrophic plans seem vulnerable to kickbacks, and should be examined to minimize that; perhaps I am wrong. Nevertheless, catastrophic was seemingly cheapest of what's available, and is certainly more flexible. If we must have mandatory health insurance – and I'm not saying we must – mandatory Catastrophic coverage sounds better than any alternative. But if we go that way, we need better studies of it.

What I Have Learned (2)

That's what I believe I have learned from the Classical Health Savings Account of 1981, and what I think will improve it still further. Essentially, that's a correction of the tax inequity, a removal of the age restrictions to make it optional at any age, and an enlargement of the deposit limits. It requires very little legislation to accomplish those three things.

But my horizons have been expanded by the reception of the original, simple proposal. So I have some suggestions for Congress to consider, for a New HSA which is an extension of the classical variety. These ideas tend to bump into other programs and require negotiation of the apparent difficulties, with resultant adjustments of other plans, originally for other purposes.

Encourage the use of index funds as sources of investment income for HSAs In this era of abnormally low interest rates, the public seems to like the substitution of common stock, even though it seems risky. I'm afraid we have learned that bonds are just as risky. But they pay considerably less, except in rare moments of "black swan" recovery from a stock market crash. Roger Ibbotson of Yale has published the long-term results of the entire stock market, which today we would equate with total market index funds. He found the results over the past century have averaged 11-12%. At a viewing distance of about three feet, regardless of many wars and stock crashes, if you had bought the whole market and forgot you had it, the average looks pretty much like a straight line. That's no guarantee it will be the same in the coming century, but it's the best guess you can make, particularly if you don't read the newspapers very often. Buy-and-hold almost becomes buy and forget.

That's the wrong risk to worry about, however. Inflation and imperfect agency are much greater risks for buy and hold. At 3% a year, inflation has reduced a dollar to a penny, in the past century. So, instead of 11-12 %, a buy-and-hold investor really only gets 8-9%, net of inflation. In addition to that, every 28-30 years he encounters a black swan stock market, loses at least 50%, and lacks the courage to buy it back at its low point. From that point forward, the market "climbs a wall of worry", and he finally buys it back just when it regains its peak.

The time-honored remedy is to buy a mixture of 60% stocks, 40% fixed income (bonds), which reduces real income to 4-6%. If we ever cure this habit, gross stock prices will probably gravitate toward paying 5-7%, gross. Unfortunately, middle-man fees and kickbacks result in the customer getting 4-6%, trying to avoid getting zero. Unfortunately, the majority of experts actually surrender somewhat less than that, and the reasonable investor simply buys index funds and forgets about them. That is, it comes out about the same, unless you get greedy, in which case most people end up losing money. For the most part, whether you win or lose, mostly has to do with where the market was when you started.

Consequently, we here advise "passive" investing, in an index mixture of total American stocks and bonds. You will do better than most people, and that's a pretty good badge of success. However, the puzzle is whether rules and regulations can improve on this result, by a tenth of a percent, here and there. Those who promise more, will probably deliver less.

Stretch out the compound interest as long as possible. Since Aristotle, it has always surprised people to find compound interest rises at the end of its term, so the longer the better is the best theory. We make three suggestions:

1. Don't buy term insurance (like most health insurance), buy whole-life. You might turn the whole business over to whole-life life insurance companies with experience in these matters, but they are private companies who can do as they please. The next-best choice is a Health Savings Account, which rolls any unspent balance over to later years, and gives it back to you at age 66. It's tax-exempt, and if you spend it on healthcare, it is doubly so.

2. Use last year of life re-insurance. People die at different ages, but the last year is usually the most costly, and it happens to everyone. If you set aside a comparatively small amount of money at birth, it will multiply 289 times at 6.5%, by the age of 84, the current average longevity. If it is transferred to Medicare, it reduces Medicare costs by at least a quarter, and Medicare really should refund a quarter of your payroll deductions as well as your Medicare premiums, maybe even more. The arithmetic is pretty complicated, but with luck it might pay for all of Medicare, except for existing debts for borrowing earlier when we ran a deficit. Furthermore. Medicare is 50% subsidized, so that has to be figured, too. Extending this subsidy to everyone is a big argument against single payer, by the way.

3. Use first year of life reinsurance. This is the reverse of the above, because the 3% of healthcare costs now thought to affect newborns is almost invariably donated by another generation. Young parents without much savings are strained to subsidize their children, so you might as well include children to the age of 21, which is 8% of healthcare costs. If you overfund Medicare by $100 at birth, it will grow by enough to subsidize grandchildren by the time grandpa dies. There are laws against perpetuities, but they limit inheritances to one lifetime, plus 21 years – plenty of time. This is a new concept which will take time to adjust to, but I can think of no other way to pre-pay a newborn infant. If you use some variant of this approach, health costs could be reduced by another 8%, for a cost of less than $100.

In closing, let me remind the reader health insurance is turning into a gigantic transfer system. The middle third of life is supporting the two-thirds, before and after. And only the last third has much sickness. People who are well don't like to subsidize those who are sick, and eventually may rebel. It's much better for young individuals to subsidize their own old age, than for one demographic group to subsidize another group of strangers. Particularly if those few who are lucky and escape much sickness, get to keep the savings for their protracted retirement.

Graphs of New HSA

T he "future value" of any sum of money is the same as the total amount accumulated in a set period of time, assuming a certain average percent of tax-exempt gain in compound interest. In matters discussed here, the future value is only generally of concern over long periods of time. Because of compounding, the future value increases at the far end. Here is a graph of the future value of almost anything at 6.5%, starting at age 80:

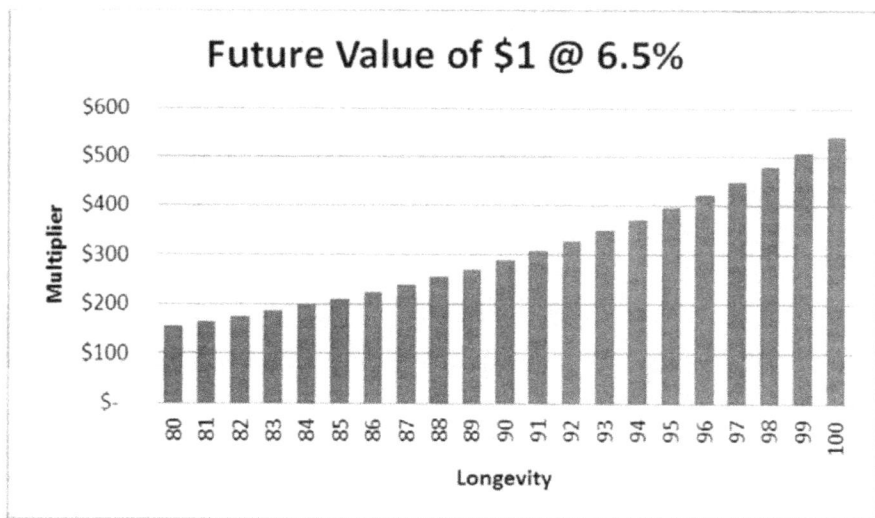

The hypothetical lifetime balance of <u>the escrow portion</u> of a New Health Savings Account would, on average, have a different shape, because the childhood portion is an inheritance at birth. It wears down over the next 20 years, so there is only a small but critical amount left over to grow during the working years, 21-66. Assuming the option is taken to fund both the first and last years this way, maximizing the income, it would look like this, assuming a longevity of 84:

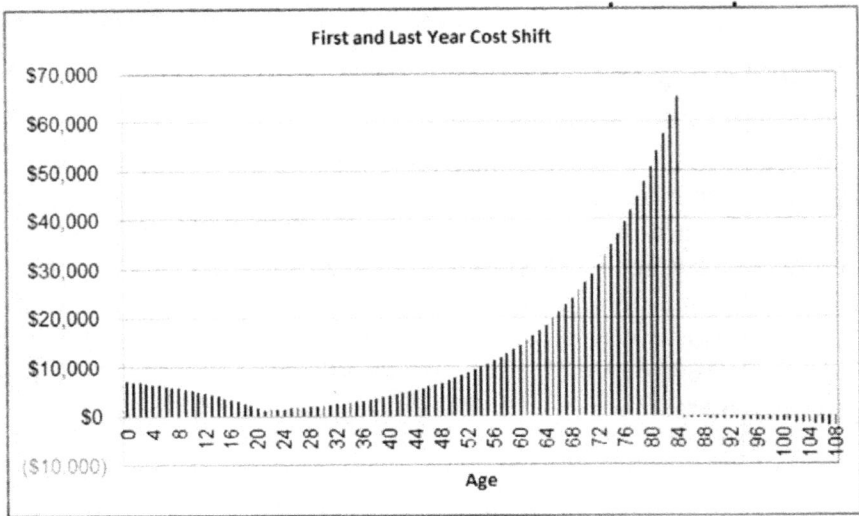

First and Last Year Cost Shift

And for age 94, the last two curves have the same overall shape, but internally result in a surplus at age 94 of about $250 a year, because the future value curve tilts upward. Remember, this may be an artifact, because there are ten extra years in which to develop new treatments to pay for:

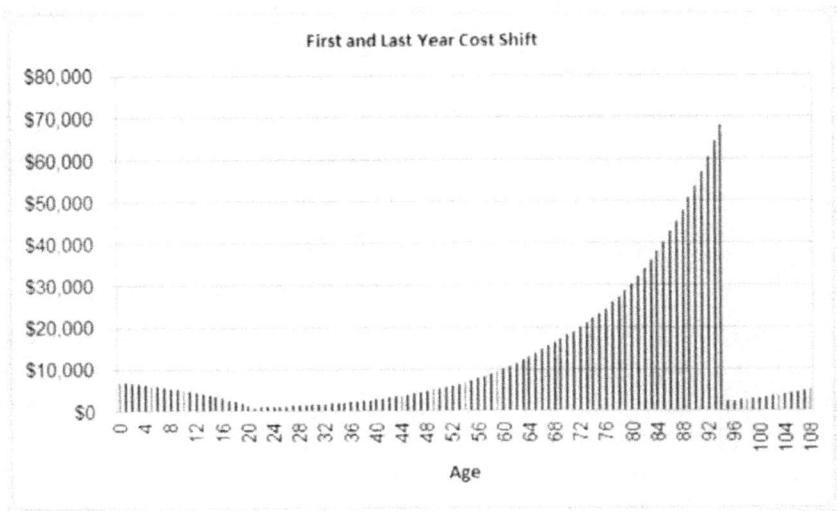

First and Last Year Cost Shift

Its component revenue would consist of $50 deposited in the account at 6.5% compound interest, every year from birth to death. That would vary with the life expectancy, which is now 84 but reasonably expected to reach 94 at some time in the next 90 years. When the contributions stop at death, the compound interest continues to accumulate for up to another 21 years, following the common law principle that a perpetuity begins after "one life, plus 21 years".

At the death of the grandfather client, the fund is nearly depleted by his first-and-last year of life reimbursements, but that payment might possibly be delayed a few months if it exactly matched his actual expenses. It could be immediate, with administrative savings, by reimbursing all primary insurance by the average cost of all last years costs. The funds left over would be comparatively small, but they would still generate income until the account is closed. However, they are a contingency cushion, and could be modified if other requirements appear.

There is a calculation perplexity in the fact that compound interest turns sharply upward, toward the end of life. Therefore, an even distribution of deaths, both longer and shorter than the mean, leads to a "profit" from the ones who live longer. Disregarding this point, the outermost limit of contributions at this level of sharply rising returns might be as much as $832,000 for a longevity of 94, and $441,000 if longevity does not increase at all. (That's assuming Obamacare joins the same system, but substitutes Catastrophic insurance for the present arrangement.) If longevity does improve, contributions of $50 a year are adequate. Longevity of less than expected (wars, famines, etc.) would mean the deposits would have to be increased. Contributions of $60 a year seem more than adequate, however.

These calculations are based on withdrawals at the time of death, for last year of life, plus first year of life, and a small surplus to spare. For the time being, the costs and revenue of Obamacare are left to that program to worry about. These accounts continue to accumulate interest during the client's 22-66 age period, but do not affect them. The thirty million uninsured are also excluded, but it would be my suggestion that they differ so much from each other, they ought to have separate programs for prisoners in jail, mentally retarded, etc.

www.ingramcontent.com/pod-product-compliance
Lightning Source LLC
Chambersburg PA
CBHW051723260326
41914CB00031B/1709/J